STORRIE™

QUANTUM WHOLISTIC HEALING™

AWAKEN YOUR JOURNEY

COMPILED BY

DR. CHRISTINE MANUKYAN

Published by STORRIE™ Publishing

Cover Design: Jennifer Rae

ISBN: 9798860688803

TABLE OF CONTENTS

ABOUT THE AUTHORS

By: Dr. Christine Manukyan, PharmD, MS

"The doctor of the future will give no medication but will instruct his patients in the care of the human frame, diet, and in the cause and prevention of disease."

– Thomas Edison, 1904

In the depths of our being lies an infinite potential for healing and transformation – a vast reservoir of untapped wisdom and energy waiting to be awakened. This book embarks on a profound exploration of the importance of **BECOMING WHOLE** and the transformative journey that awaits us through the realm of **QUANTUM WHOLISTIC HEALING™**.

When you make the decision to stop allowing fear to get in your way, you unlock the potential to change your life and the lives of those around you. When I left my job during the global pandemic in 2020 and started my entrepreneurial journey as a Functional Medicine practitioner and business coach, I visualized creating a tribe of clinicians who believed in **WHOLE-BODY HEALTH** using holistic principles just as much as I did. I pictured the ways our lives would change forever as we stepped into a new chapter of our lives. I knew that it was possible, and I knew my tribe was out there somewhere.

The authors you will meet within the pages of this book are my tribe, who are here to make an impact on world health with Wholistic Wellness™. At STORRIE Institute™, we define Wholistic Wellness™ as the practice of returning to our natural state of health by adopting a lifestyle that supports the body's innate ability to heal and thrive.

In this book you will read about the authors who are the courageous healthcare professionals and coaches who have chosen to step out of a life riddled with burnout and into a purpose-filled life where balance is truly possible. Together, these authors are empowering others to reach their health goals without pharmaceuticals and to find real answers through using Wholistic Wellness Coaching™.

Within the interconnected tapestry of our mind, body, and spirit lies the key to unlocking the true essence of our existence. As we embrace the quantum principles that govern the universe, we embark on a sacred quest to discover the limitless possibilities of self-healing and growth. This journey within not only promises to mend our fragmented selves but also unveils the profound interconnectedness with the cosmic dance of life, empowering us to step into a reality where profound healing and self-discovery converge harmoniously. So, let us venture forth with an open heart and a curious mind, for within the depths of our consciousness, the journey towards wholeness and awakening awaits.

This tribe of clinicians and coaches have gone first and have realized that it's time we create the **WHOLISTIC WELLNESS REVOLUTION™** and change lives around the world using the healing modalities that have existed forever – natural and holistic medicine. The stories the authors are sharing will serve as proof of their resilient spirits, and our hope is that you will be inspired by their journeys to take action and create the life you are worthy of living. This collaborative book is evidence that anyone can reclaim their power, unlock their impact, surrender, awaken their healing journey, and unleash their full potential.

These authors have become my best friends and colleagues. We laugh together, we cry together, and we always have each other's back. Each author came into my life for a distinct reason. Individually, they have gone through a lot, and until this moment, their experiences have been locked away within them, just waiting to be honored and shared. Now is the time for their stories to be unleashed and their impact to be felt across the world.

The main goal of ***Quantum Wholistic Healing™: Awaken Your Journey*** is to honor the stories shared so that their legacies can live on and help you unleash your own truth, surrender, and continue to heal and grow from within. They all bring in their unique voices and gifts into STORRIE Institute™, and for that, I am forever grateful.

This is my tribe, and together we are **CREATING THE NEW GOLD STANDARD OF CARE.** At STORRIE Institute™, we are on track to create a Doctoral Degree in Wholistic Wellness™ that believes in transformative power of **WHOLISTIC HEALING**.

Live your passion,

Dr. Christine Manukyan | www.storrie.co
Founder & CEO: STORRIE Institute™ & STORRIE Wellness™
Host: STORRIE™ Podcast

FOREWORD

By: Britt Gregorio

"Let go of the stories that keep you small."

– Aggie Lal

Impossible. That one word holds so much meaning, and for every unique person, it's vastly different.

Humans have been programmed to accept defeat when a situation or circumstance is deemed impossible. But what would happen if you surrounded yourself with the thought that nothing is ever truly impossible?

What would you be capable of? What would that feel like? How free would you feel?

Whenever life puts us in situations that are hard and "impossible," doubt and fear seep in. We tell ourselves the narrative of, "That level of success is not possible," or, "It's impossible to change careers, I'm too old," and even, "Healing my body is impossible."

We have all been there once or twice, right? Feeding ourselves the narrative of having to stay in a box because we tell ourselves to, or society tells us to.

It's one thing to tell yourself that you've got this and you'll overcome … eventually. But it's profoundly different when you immerse yourself in knowing that you can do and achieve anything you want in life.

You can make that change you've always wanted, you can lose the weight, you can overcome illness, you can find the answers, you can have the success. You, my beautiful friend, are fully capable of shutting out impossibilities from your being.

In my experience, expanding into the holistic and Functional Medicine realm eliminates barriers for impossibilities. There is so much goodness to learn about different healing modalities.

Over the span of 15 years, I've found that healing the mind, body, and soul provides freedom, a freedom to really know what your inner self and physical body wants, and the means to provide it.

I won't bore you with all the details, but there was a time in my life when I was told I'd never walk again. Then I was told I'd never have kids. After my first son was born, he battled a seven-year illness I was told was incurable. As I got older and began my journey of entrepreneurship, people around me laughed and said it was impossible with all that was going on in my life. As I currently write this foreword, my middle son is having difficulty with worsening autism and possibly mental health issues. I've been told by several specialists that it's impossible to help him without hospitalization.

An important piece of my background is that as a child, I was a rebel. I knew in my soul that I was different. As I entered adulthood and my own physical health declined, that rebel mentality kicked in and ultimately led me into holistic practices.

It took 10 years for me to walk freely again after a severe injury. I did go on to have three extraordinary boys. My firstborn was healed from his illness. I became a successful business owner, copywriting for purpose-driven brands around the world. My special middle guy is finally going to get the help he needs from a holistic center in New York City.

Most of my life was surrounded by the impossible. When a doctor, or family member, or lawyer told me all was lost, that inner rebel emerged and said, "Watch me make it happen."

There is nothing overly special about me. I wasn't born into a wealthy family. For many years as a single mom, we lived in poverty. I never had a backup plan. What I do have are my fiery rebel problem-solving skills and holistic background. Today, I'm simply a human who rights wrongs and laughs at all impossible things.

Once you practice banishing fear and expectation (and it is a daily practice), you feel a strong sense of wholeness. Awakening your mind, body, and soul opens you up to what can be: a sea of possibilities.

The authors of this book have taken a stand against the impossible. They have been called by holistic practices and Functional Medicine to elevate healing. They have released the blockages holding them back and refuse to settle. The stories that you will experience reading this book are invaluable.

It is my deepest wish that you allow this book to fill you with awareness, hope, and a deep sense of what can be.

Remember, things are only impossible if you allow them to be.

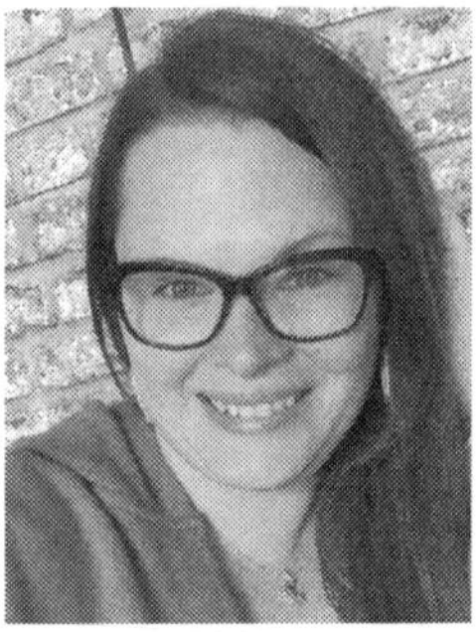

ABOUT BRITT GREGORIO

Brittany Gregorio is a copy & content writer known to write from the heart. She has written for dozens of brands across the country, and her articles have been in prestigious publications. Her heart-centered intentionality allows her to convert in a big way for her clients.

Prior to her writing career, she immersed herself in yogic practices and energetic healing to overcome physical and emotional trauma. After becoming a Yoga & Meditation Teacher, & Reiki Practitioner, she knew her purpose was to combine her love of yoga & healing with writing. Working with entrepreneurs in the yoga, energetic, and holistic space sets her soul on fire.

Brittany is known as a free spirit while keeping things real and overcoming the impossible. She believes the key to success is to lean into what makes you uniquely you. She spent many years ignoring her gifts, but she fully embraces them today while running a successful writing business. Elevating her education is a must and just as this book goes to publishing she's currently completing her Ayurvedic Practitioner Certification.

https://linktr.ee/brittanygregorio | britt@thecopychick.com | IG: @brittany.gregorio

BREATHE. HEAL. SURRENDER.

By: Dr. Christine Manukyan, PharmD, MS

"Healing is not a destination; it's a quantum journey of self-discovery, love, and acceptance, leading us back to the wholeness we've always been."

– Dr. Christine Manukyan

Each one of us carries within the innate capacity for transformation and growth, a seed of potential waiting to bloom. **Quantum Wholistic Healing™** teaches us that the mind, body, and spirit are inseparable, and true healing is achieved when we address all three as one. This chapter of my story embarks on an extraordinary expedition – a quest to unleash the healing power that resides within us and embrace the essence of **Wholistic Wellness™.**

On average, we take 20,000 breaths per day. That's 20,000 times you can put a pause on your hectic day, connect with your breath by sitting or laying down for a minute, maybe even meditating for five minutes, then moving on with your day. What if you are told you have five years to live before you take your last breath? How would you spend your time on Earth? Will you be focusing on things that don't matter and are stressing you out, or would you find time to spend with your loved ones, laughing together and creating memories? This was what I was told in 2015, something I didn't want to hear.

In 2020, a year filled with endless unknowns, I trusted my intuition and walked away from the career I was building for over 20 years. On my 40th birthday, I became a corporate dropout. I was exhausted from the demands of working full-time and homeschooling (schools were closed due to the global pandemic), not to mention trying to find child care when my husband and I were working. I spent the majority of 2020 on the front lines as a hospital pharmacist in one of the busiest hospitals in the nation. By August of 2020, I had enough. I trusted the universe to guide me, and I made the decision to leave my job and reclaim my life by diving headfirst into the world of Functional Medicine and entrepreneurship, instead. I was no longer willing to accept the fact that the medications I was handing to my patients were only a temporary solution to their deep-rooted problems. I knew that there was a better way, and I was willing to do whatever it took to help people find real healing. This decision led to the first chapter in my pursuit to rewrite my story.

My decision to leave was the first step in unleashing the story that was trapped inside my visionary mind for far too long. Within a year of becoming a corporate dropout, I celebrated my very first multiple six-figure month. I had changed the narrative of "I'm just a pharmacist" to "I am Dr. Christine Manukyan, and I am leading the Wholistic Wellness Revolution™ through STORRIE Institute™."

What is Wholistic Wellness™?

At both of my companies, STORRIE Institute™ and STORRIE Wellness™, we define Wholistic Wellness™ as the practice of returning to our natural state of health by adopting a lifestyle that supports the body's innate ability to heal and thrive. Wholistic Wellness™ includes Functional

Medicine, Integrative Medicine, Lifestyle Medicine, Ayurvedic Medicine, Chinese Medicine, Orthomolecular Medicine, Energy Healing, Nutrition, and Herbalism.

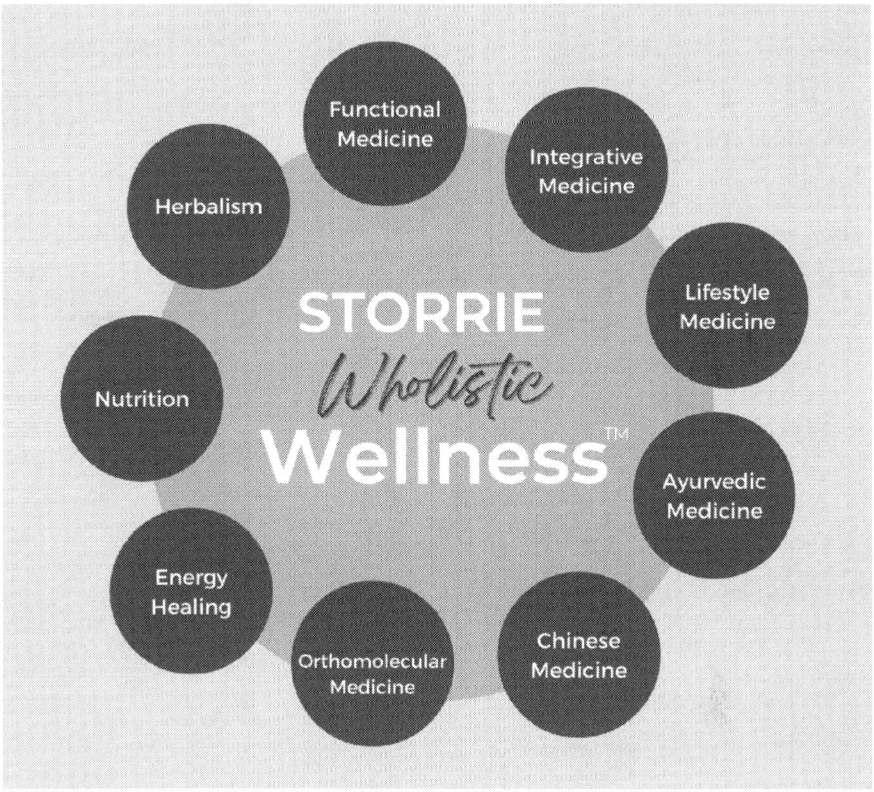

Big shift, isn't it? Well, I would be lying if I said it was a smooth and easy transition from just Functional Medicine to Wholistic Wellness™, but with grit, hard work, determination, and allowing my breath and my intuition to guide me, it is possible! And I know that for a fact: Wholistic Wellness Coaching™ is the future of healthcare with a vision to create a Doctoral Degree in Wholistic Wellness™.

Our stories are an evolutionary process. We become who we are through our childhood experiences and the choices we make as we grow up. I was a first-generation Armenian American. At just 16 years old, I moved to the United States, excited about the future ahead. One of the first things I had to get used to was the "American diet." I didn't know about things like processed food, GMOs, artificial colors and sweeteners, chemicals, preservatives, pesticides and all the other stuff that is often found in our food. When I was growing up, I remember my grandparents always using home remedies whenever we caught a cold or flu, and they rarely used any medications to treat anything. Organic food was all I knew because, back home during the '80s, that's all we had. Organic fresh food was our nutrition and our medicine. I drank water from the water faucet without thinking twice about if it had any additional chemicals, and I would eat butter every day without worrying about cholesterol. We would walk everywhere, occasionally take public transportation, but I was constantly active and moving my body because that was just part of our culture. We shopped at farmers markets and ate fruits and vegetables that were in season. Looking back, I realize we grew up with an ideal healthy lifestyle that was easy to take for granted.

It didn't take long for me to experience the effects of the crappy and cheap fast food I consumed as a teenager living in America. The more I ate, the more I realized how sick my body was becoming. I found myself gaining weight, struggling with energy, and having a hard time focusing. This was not normal for me. Ultimately, my diet and lifestyle were affecting my mood, self-esteem, and self-worth. My family couldn't afford to purchase organic food, as we were living paycheck to paycheck and received government assistance at the time. We could only afford cheap fast food that had absolutely no nutritional value and was just filled with crap.

If you grew up in the United States, you probably know exactly what I'm talking about. In fact, if you were raised in this Western culture, you may only know the American lifestyle as your norm. As someone who was new to this environment, however, I had no idea of the long-term health issues this traditional "American diet" can cause. Growing up as a teenager, I was just trying to just fit in. I acclimated to this new lifestyle, and little did I know, this would lead me to a variety of health challenges when I entered my 30s. The bad eating and exercise habits continued through my time in undergraduate and pharmacy school. I remember drinking three to four cans of diet soda each day, adding five to seven packets of Splenda® into my coffee, and eating ramen noodles filled with soy, sodium, and GMOs. I would think to myself, "I am young, I don't have any health issues, so why not?" And when you add stress on top of a poor lifestyle, you may not know it, but you are speeding up the natural aging process.

Like many others, I was trading my health for potential wealth, and was focused on achieving the "American dream." I worked hard throughout pharmacy school, and graduated with honors while being class president and leader of several organizations. I was also working part-time at a retail pharmacy, but to be honest, it was rough. After graduating from Nova Southeastern University College of Pharmacy, I found myself constantly chasing the next big thing. For me, this looked like moving to Ohio from Florida and living alone for the first time while completing a two-year residency at The Ohio State University Medical Center. I was also working on my master's degree in Health-System Pharmacy Administration. Needless to say, there was a lot on my plate, and my personal health was not a priority at the time.

Within months of graduating from residency, I married my high school sweetheart, who also happened to become a hospital pharmacist. We quickly started our family and had two children. Having back-to-back pregnancies while working full time at the hospital also took a huge toll on my health. I was still chasing the next big thing. I was chasing after promotions at work and chasing after the unrealistic idea that I could be the "perfect" wife and mom. In no time, I found myself living my life on autopilot and again, it took a huge toll on my body. While I was climbing the leadership ladder at work, I was slowly dying inside. Plus, back-to-back pregnancies caused more weight gain and spiraled my health completely out of control. As a new mother, I was focused on my family, work, and others. I forgot all about self-love and self-care. I was morbidly obese, and saw my health declining as my career was seemingly blooming. My energy was almost nonexistent, however, and I was unable to be fully present with my kids. I knew I could not continue like this, but I didn't know how much of a dire health situation I had gotten myself into.

In 2015, at 35 years old, I scheduled my annual checkup. At this appointment, I was told by my primary care physician that I was going to have a heart attack in the next five years if I continued with the lifestyle I had been living. I mean, who wants to hear they are going to take their last breath by age 40? That was scary, but the truth was I was morbidly obese, extremely burnt out, had high cholesterol, low energy, insomnia, brain fog, and unexplained inflammation, and was under never-ending stress. I can honestly say I was a hot mess mamma who was just trying to take care of my two little ones while also working full time at a management level, which was increasingly more stressful. Ironically from the outside, I looked fine, and I definitely didn't look "sick."

During that office visit with my primary care doctor, I was given a pill to lower my cholesterol, and I was told to go "lose some weight." Nothing was explained, and I wasn't given any guidance on how to go about losing weight or if there were any other options out there to help to improve my health. As a pharmacist, I knew I was just being prescribed a toxic pill that was known to have many side effects. I was stunned and humiliated. I blamed myself, and kept thinking, "I should have known better." I was confused, and felt as if I had lost part of my identity.

I walked out of that 10-minute doctor's appointment so disappointed. Not only was I told I was going to die soon if I didn't make changes right away, but I had also waited six months to even see the doctor, and once I arrived, I waited over an hour before the doctor came into the room. My experience from start to finish was terrible. After the appointment, I sat in my car crying, and began to feel increasingly more anxious about how I was going to fix this. I was overwhelmed and terrified at the thought of not being around to watch my children grow. I just knew there had to be a better way to reclaim my health without the toxic little pill I had been told to take.

This appointment had me spinning. I wanted to know why, as a patient, I was left to feel this way. Why wasn't my doctor asking me how I felt about taking this prescription? Why wasn't she having a conversation with me about what else I could do to lower my cholesterol? After all, according to my labs, it was only my cholesterol that was the problem. This also caused me to wonder why my doctor didn't even ask me how I was. If I had been asked how I was really feeling, I would have shared that I was burnt out, overwhelmed, and overall, was not ok. The reality is, routine labs don't always tell the story of how a person is feeling, they just don't.

Without even realizing it, I had been sitting in my car for over an hour thinking about what had just happened. I had to gather my strength and pull myself together so I could drive home and face the reality that I wasn't prepared to face. As I was driving, I kept praying and manifesting for someone to come into my life who could help me. I needed someone who could be my accountability buddy to help me lose weight without starving myself. I had failed so many diets in the past, and I was tired of the unsuccessful dieting attempts that led me nowhere near being "healthy." I knew a decision needed to be made, so I started researching and gave myself time to discover a better way to lower my cholesterol and lose weight.

It was time for me to make a decision that would change my life forever. The choice I faced was either to settle and just take the pill, or I could challenge myself to look for an alternative. Spoiler alert, I chose option two. I focused my energy looking for alternative ways to heal my body. Taking care of my health suddenly became my top priority. After several weeks of searching, I found a solution. My friend and colleague introduced me to the realm of holistic health and led me toward receiving the best Mother's Day present I could have ever given myself. On Mother's Day in 2015 (May 11, 2015), I committed to rewriting my story in order to become the best version of myself. This season of my life was the beginning of something big. If my life was a book, 2015 would be the foreword – *Choosing To Rewrite My Story.*

This commitment led me straight in the direction of Functional Medicine. I soon began focusing more on uncovering the root cause of my failing health and relearning how to use food as medicine. I realized my health was interconnected with my highly stressful career, so I made the decision to step down from my management position to work in hopes of bringing down my stress levels. This was a very hard decision to make, especially since this was the first time after all these years I would no longer be "the boss." I knew this was all a part of rewriting my story and reclaiming life, though, so it was time for me to focus on what mattered the most to me – my health and my family. Putting aside my ego and title to focus on a healthy lifestyle was incredibly challenging, but worth it. For the first time in my life, I had to really ask myself, "How am I doing?" Being "fine" or just "OK" was not good enough for me. I needed time to go back to the basics. For over 16 years, I lived an unhealthy lifestyle, so it would take determination to not fall back into the same habits I had become accustomed to.

Fast-forward six months, and I was at a follow-up appointment with my same primary care doctor. My doctor wanted to make sure my labs were OK because I was supposed to start taking the cholesterol-lowering medication. I intentionally didn't say anything about not taking the medication, as I wanted to see if the lifestyle changes I had made would reflect in my lab work. I can remember this moment so clearly. My doctor walked in the room and told me, "I think there is a lab error, we might have to redo your labs. Your labs are normal, and I don't think the medication works that fast." I smiled at her and said, "There was no lab error, what you're looking at is the power of using food as medicine, incorporating adaptogens for stress management and natural energy, cellular cleansing, and intermittent fasting." I had also lost 35 pounds of toxic visceral fat, the fat that was surrounding my organs and causing all the health issues I was previously experiencing. I then started to share with her what changes I had been making over the last six months. My doctor was so impressed and asked me to send her more information so she could share it with her other patients. She even asked me if I was OK with her connecting me to others who would like to learn more about a holistic lifestyle. I got the green light from her to continue what I was doing. That one decision to change my health without pharmaceuticals and instead incorporate Functional Medicine became the catalyst of my life transformation journey, which later on became my passion, mission, and calling.

After experiencing my own health transformation using Wholistic Wellness™, I realized the power that comes from making better decisions and how one decision can transform your entire life. My desire to chase the next big thing never went away, but instead of limiting myself to chase success through my job and unrealistic societal expectations, I decided to chase true success that started from within: within my very own body. Over time, I went on to lose over 100 pounds through intermittent fasting, exercise, and incorporating Functional Medicine practices into my daily routine. I even experienced a boost of self-confidence that allowed me to step out on stage as a fitness competitor (bodybuilder). I stepped on stage as the real-life Wonder Woman, in order to empower other women to say "Yes!" to themselves and be an example of what's possible when you take consistent action. I also went on to run the LA Marathon on March 8, 2020 – the very year that I would also turn 40. Mamma didn't have a heart attack like the doctor said – instead she ran a 26-mile marathon! When I crossed the finish line, I felt like I was the success story I had always hoped to become!

I became my first "client," using a holistic lifestyle to reach health goals, without realizing that my experiences would turn into my career just a few years later. For a while, I was still doing this as a "side gig" as I was still working full-time in the hospital and was not yet looking for an exit strategy. Well, that didn't last too long before I hit another rock bottom and found myself in the same exact place, confused and overwhelmed. I was, again, asking myself, "Is this it? Is this what I am meant to be doing for the rest of my life until I retire?" I felt so out of balance and unsettled because deep down, I knew I was meant for so much more. I just didn't know what it was going to look like until one day I heard a podcast that changed my life.

My commute used to take over two hours a day, most of which was spent sitting in traffic. I would often listen to podcasts to kill time. One evening, as I was driving home and trying to keep my eyes open after a very stressful evening shift at the hospital, I turned on a podcast where a

Nurse Practitioner was sharing her story about how she went from traditional medicine into Functional Medicine and now has her own online practice. This happened to be the same day I was introduced to a master coach who worked alongside one of the most highly recognized business and life strategists in the nation. As I was listening to these women and their stories, I felt like they were speaking straight to my soul. I heard terms like "time freedom," "working from home," and "making a real impact in the world" for the very first time. I was eager to learn more, and started asking questions like, "How does an online practice work? What training and certifications are needed? Will the California Board of Pharmacy really allow me to have my own practice?" I mean, a million questions passed through my mind. These were all questions that I had never thought of asking myself, so it felt strange to even think about starting my own business. This was a huge investment, and I quickly started to question my ability to achieve these dreams of mine. The thought "What happens if I fail?" was top of mind.

It was January 2020, and something inside me switched on and suddenly my soul was on fire. I just knew this was going to be my year, no matter what. I knew that in order to make big, bold decisions, I needed to be surrounded by mentors and people who cheer me on and help me achieve my dreams. I needed a tribe that would elevate me so I could unleash my full potential! I invested in my very first personal development program with Karissa Kouchis, and became a founding member of her tribe, Unleash Her Power Within (UHPW).

I spent all year manifesting and preparing to leave my job by my 40th birthday. I dreamed and visualized creating my own Functional Medicine legacy. Like many people who make a pivot, I was so scared. I started doubting myself and questioning if I really knew enough to open my own practice. I was second-guessing myself and wondering if I made the right decision in hiring a business coach, someone I had just met. Then I remembered why I hired my business coach in the first place. I did this because my *why* was so strong. I no longer wanted to choose between my health, my family, and my career, and I knew it was possible to have freedom in all of these areas of life.

Once I was done with making excuses and waiting for the "right time," I got out of my own way and got to work. In March 2020, the global pandemic quickly proved that I was making the right investments and decisions for my life. The world was changing so quickly. Overnight, telemedicine and online virtual practice became the new normal. I quickly realized how much I had to learn and how fast I needed to implement everything I had been learning. As a clinical pharmacist, I was trained in the acute care hospital setting for 13 years, and now I had to shift my focus to preventative medicine using Functional Medicine. There was a tight deadline to get things in order because I was set to launch my practice in May. There was a lot on my plate, but I stayed laser-focused on my vision, and nothing could distract me. I was like one of those race horses with their side blinders on, running in one lane, fast and with intention. I learned how to own my worth and charge for my services and my consultations. All of this to become a business owner, Functional Medicine practitioner, and coach.

There was an opportunity in my profession as a pharmacist that many haven't thought about. I saw an opportunity for growth and an exit strategy if the pandemic was going to last longer than anticipated. Creating my own virtual Functional Medicine practice during the pandemic became my goal so I could fully walk away from the corporate world. I finally figured out the solution to my health, lifestyle, and career problems. I could now work from home as my own boss, without sacrificing my income, and I could do all this by launching my own virtual Functional

Medicine practice. Once again, I felt so accomplished. I created something, without knowing exactly how it would happen, and let the desire to rewrite my story guide my way. I knew I would have many challenges along the way, and I was OK with that. It was a bold decision, and it was something that the real-life Wonder Woman would do, so I did it.

On May 11, 2020, I launched my Functional Medicine practice. Crazy enough, this was exactly five years after starting my own health transformation journey and being a health coach. For a while, I continued working limited hours on the weekends at the hospital, in addition to my job. I realized that our child-care situation wasn't perfect, but we made it work as long as we could. Then, one day in late May, I was informed that my work schedule could not be accommodated any longer and that I needed to go back to work full-time starting in June. Telling our kids that we had to hire a nanny, a complete stranger from an agency, so I could go back to work, was one of the hardest days of my life. Both kids cried and asked questions like, "Why are you leaving us? What if this person hurts us? What if we get sick? Why is work more important than us?" I cried as I tried to comfort them, saying things like, "Everything will be OK" and, "We will get through this together." It was so hard, and I couldn't sleep for many days in a row. I had to choose to go back to work, as working from home was not an option at the time, and I wasn't fully ready to leave my job. In my mind, I was still waiting for the perfect time to leave. I didn't have the mindset that was necessary in order to make big changes right at that moment. It was so hard, knowing I had no other options but to leave the kids and go back to work full-time.

Even though I had technically launched my Functional Medicine practice at the time, it was only a "side gig." I quickly realized that having one foot in my own practice and one foot in my corporate career was not serving anybody well, especially myself and my family. I was only doing a half-ass job, and was not able to generate the amount of income (or impact) needed to turn my side-gig into a full-time job, not while still working full-time as a pharmacist, at least. A month or so into trying to balance both, I couldn't tolerate the pain any longer. I had to make a decision and move forward. There are always more decisions to make. Knowing when and how to make them is the most important part of implementing change.

At this point, I was hitting yet another rock bottom. In July 2020, I decided to attend a huge virtual event, Unleash The Power Within, hosted by the same highly recognized business and life strategist, Tony Robbins, whose tribe I was already a part of. My kids saw me go through a transformational breakthrough. They heard me speak my goals out loud and knew that I was working to find a way to work from home so I would be able to be home with them. This event changed my life. It was there that I gained clarity of what I wanted to do. In large part, this was because I was surrounded by others who were hungry for growth as much as I was. I broke through my fears of failure by physically breaking a board in half! On one side of the board, I wrote "Fear of Failure" and on the other side I wrote, "I am unstoppable, I am Wonder Woman." During this virtual event, I listened as person after person told their stories of passion and drive towards making a real difference in this world and supporting others along the way.

I had finally gained clarity about my calling and got the guts to pursue my purpose to help others rewrite their stories to become the best version of themselves, just like I was doing! This realization came at the perfect time in my life. I finally realized that in order to truly rewrite my story, I had to put two feet into my Functional Medicine practice and work through the uncomfortable feelings associated with the risk.

Come August 2020, my kids were starting online school again, just like the majority of kids in the nation. Knowing I had no reliable child care, I made the terrifying decision to take a huge pay cut and walk away from my full-time job. This was the most stable job I had ever had, as I had been working there for over a decade. Letting go of my job allowed me to focus 100 percent on my family and in my new practice. I walked away from my six-figure career and reputation as a leading pharmacist to step into the space of entrepreneurship. It was a risk, but it was also the goal that I had been manifesting all year.

The pandemic made me realize just how quickly our lives can change and how much we can do to change our lives if we have a burning desire to pursue our purpose. Walking away from security and moving forward without the answers totally goes against my life-long training of doing the research before taking action. It was scary, but also so exciting. And it all just felt so right, and there was finally space in my life for me to relax and enjoy time with my family.

After leaving my job, I spent an entire month slowing down and catching up with life. I will never forget the feeling of waking up the following morning and feeling free! I felt like 1,000 pounds of weight was lifted off of my shoulders. I wasn't rushing anywhere, I wasn't hitting the snooze on the alarm over and over. I didn't have to be anywhere at a particular time. I was finally able to just be present with my family. That morning, I became a full-time mom for the very first time. It actually happened to be a very special day, when I had the privilege of witnessing my son receive his black belt in Tae Kwon Do. I sat back, thinking about how I had been a part-time mom for over a decade and missed out on so many milestones, but that was no longer my heartbreaking reality. Witnessing my son earn his black belt was the best feeling this mamma could have ever asked for. We both accomplished something that was scary and took a lot of grit to accomplish. It was hard work, but we did it!

The reason I am sharing all these details is that they each played a key part in my story. We are often told things like, "Everything will work out" and, "Everything happens for a reason." I believe this is true, even though we may not see or understand it at the moment. Remember, my health transformation started in 2015 after hearing my doctor tell me I would have a heart attack within five years if I didn't start taking a pill and losing weight. Honestly, if my doctor didn't use those words to "scare" me, I wouldn't have taken my health as seriously as I did. I wouldn't have immediately looked for a better way to take care of my health. I wouldn't have found holistic health. I wouldn't have found my tribe and community who continue to inspire me every single day. Everything really does happen for a reason, and at just the right time in our lives. Painful moments are often the puzzle pieces of life that come together to create a beautiful masterpiece later in life.

If you are experiencing rejection from something you have worked so hard for, consider it to be a redirection towards your next big thing. **You never know when your detour will take you to your destiny**. I have been rejected several times, two of which I will never forget. First, I was rejected from multiple pharmacy schools in California, only to be put on a waitlist with no hope of getting in. Then, I moved all the way to Florida, only to find out that same day that one of the schools in California actually decided to accept me. Frustration and confusion could have set in, but instead, I knew there was a reason I was meant to go to pharmacy school in Florida. If I hadn't made the scary decision to move to Florida, I would never have met some of my best friends. Second, there is a reason I was rejected from a position I applied for within my pharmacy department. If I had started with that position, it would have kept me in the same place for many years instead of stepping into something new – my real purpose. It's no secret that life will suck sometimes. At times, it may seem as though life is unfair, and to be completely honest, sometimes it is. Don't let that distract you from the lessons you are meant to learn though and trust the path you are being redirected to. Stay the course, your course, and all really will work out in the end.

When I made the conscious decision to slow down and take the entire month of September off, I began manifesting and visualizing how I would be spending my days, where I would focus my energy, and how I could serve those who need me the most. When I first launched my online practice, I focused on helping women lose weight, detox their bodies, gain energy, and reduce stress. Those were my main pillars of health that I knew for a fact would change their lives. In addition to these pillars, I offered Functional Medicine-specific lab testing to take the guesswork out in order to focus on the root cause. I knew there were a lot of women who were struggling and desperately looking for solutions that I could offer.

Part of me kept holding back from going all in and scaling my clinical services up because I found myself having dozens of conversations with other burnt-out pharmacists who were in the exact same shoes as I was. They were also stuck between two worlds, choosing between their career that no longer fulfilled them and their families who needed them. Hearing my colleagues go through the same pain and struggle, I knew I had to provide them with a solution and help them out in a way that nobody else has yet to offer. At this time, I had many tearful conversations with colleagues and other pharmacists who wanted to know how they could also reclaim their lives. Many of these people were moms who were in very similar shoes as I was. They were stressed, overwhelmed, and overworked, while also not making the impact on their patients that they desperately longed for. These conversations made me realize that I needed to invest in my own growth, so I could show up for these men and women and be able to lead as their mentor.

After five years of health coaching and changing 300+ lives, I knew that I was still being called to expand my reach beyond health coaching. The conversations I was having with other clinicians led me to experience a vision of leading other clinicians away from a life riddled with corporate burnout and outlandish expectations to a life of freedom that, I knew first-hand, was possible. After more months of research and business coaching, I accepted the first member into STORRIE Institute™ (formerly called Functional Medicine Business Academy™) on November 11, 2020. Our clinicians are highly educated individuals, and coaching was just the beginning of what they needed to gain the confidence and knowledge in order to open their own Wholistic Wellness™ practices and become a Certified Functional Medicine Specialist™.

Looking back, I realize that I didn't do everything perfectly, but I am glad I've been able to learn from my mistakes so that I can help equip others to do things differently. When I first started my business, there were lots of people I took advice from. Some of it was great, but just not for me and my business. Here's the lesson from that: You don't know what you don't know. Not many people have walked the path before me in this industry, so I just pulled as much as I could from the resources and support that was available. I am thankful for everything that I've gone through because now I am able to also pull from my experiences to help serve my clinicians and equip them to be better prepared when they are starting their own practices and begin working with clients. I learned a lot of things the hard way. Nonetheless, I made strides forward with every decision I made. Good and bad decisions have only made the foundation of my business stronger and more able to withstand the challenges to come.

Through the conversations, coaching, and feedback I have received over the years, we are finally at a pivotal point of combining all that has already been built through STORRIE Institute™, with something entirely new. There is a clear need to revolutionize how clinicians and coaches are able to practice healthcare, and I am committed to paving the path for them to make the kind of impact we all set out to make when pursuing the field of medicine. I am excited to announce that we officially not only offer a certification program to become a **Certified STORRIE Wholistic Wellness Coach™** but also have created **STORRIE Community Mastermind™** for clinicians and coaches who believe in our mission, impacting millions of lives with Wholistic Wellness™. For more information on how you can get certified as a wellness coach or join our community mastermind, visit our website at www.storrieinstitute.com.

Each and every one of us has the responsibility to control where we choose to place our energy and attention. If we choose to focus on revolutionizing how patients are being taken care of, we will learn the skills needed to accomplish that vision. Everything is energy, and our intuition and our breath are here to guide us. I am speaking from experience as I witnessed my own life transform in front of my eyes as I let my breath be my guide. Recently I became a Certified Breathwork Practitioner, then completed Board Certification in Reiki, Clinical Hypnotherapy, Neuro Linguistic Programing (NLP), Emotional Freedom Technique (EFT), Time Technique, Gene Testing (i.e. Nutrigenetics, Nutrigenomics, and Pharmacogenomics), Sound Bowl Healing, Chakra Healing, and Life & Success Coaching. I manifested all these changes highlighted in my story using breathwork and energy healing modalities. I encourage all of you to do the same. Slow down, tap into your subconscious mind, release all the blocks that have been holding you back, manifest your dream life, step into that magical experience like it already exists, and **Let Your Breath Be Your Guide™**.

As a successful entrepreneur, I have invested over $250K working with business coaches who have mentored me to launch and scale both of my companies. However, something was missing. I got the strategy I needed, but I hit rock bottom going through burnout as an entrepreneur, even thinking of shutting down my businesses. My health was starting to decline. I gained over 60 lbs in three years. This is when I knew I had to make a change in the coaching industry. As a wellness practitioner and business coach who teaches energy healing modalities, I have created a program fostering a holistic approach to entrepreneurship. The **Energetics of Entrepreneurship™** program is designed to empower entrepreneurs who are scaling their businesses from six to seven figures and are facing burnout. This transformative program combines business mentoring and energy healing modalities to help participants regulate their nervous system, releasing mental and emotional blocks, and build thriving business while rediscovering the joy in their entrepreneurial journey. If you are an entrepreneur looking for a community that blends business strategies with energy healing techniques, you may apply to work with me on our website www.storrie.co.

I started this healing journey in 2022, and started off going to Bali and really tapping into my breath to guide me. Deep down I knew there is more to this healing journey and I hadn't experienced it yet until I attended Dr. Joe Dispenza's week-long meditation retreat in 2023. This event changed my life in so many ways. I learned that in order for me to heal, I must change. Dr. Joe showed me what's possible when you meditate in order to change, instead of meditating to heal. I didn't understand the difference until I experienced what he was saying. During the week-long meditation retreat, he challenged us to pick an area of our life that we want to change, something that is no longer serving us, and let go of those feelings that are energetically bringing us down. After deep thinking, I knew I had to focus on **FORGIVENESS**, forgiving myself, forgiving those who have hurt me, forgiving those who have lied to me, forgiving those who have taken advantage of me, forgiveness for my dad. Focusing on forgiveness during our meditations was magical. I learned how to forgive and replace all the anger, frustration, betrayal, and all those negative feelings with love, abundance, joy, and gratitude. During these meditations, I changed who I was becoming, and as I changed, I was able to **HEAL**.

Coming back from the meditation retreat, I found the strength to visit my dad after 10-plus years of no contact, and for the very first time, my kids not only learned they have a grandpa but also came to meet him with me. I can't explain how FREE I felt, letting go of the negative emotions towards my dad and everyone who has hurt me, and replacing them with love and gratitude. This would not have been possible if I didn't **SURRENDER** to the outcome during the meditation retreat. To learn more about my experience, I invite you to listen to STORRIE™ Podcast Episode 118: Meditation Retreat With Dr. Joe Dispenza.

As a Wholistic Wellness Coach™, I continue to add wellness services that are not only aligned with what my heart desires, but also are the desires from those around me, from my community. I am so excited to offer the **QUANTUM WHOLISTIC HEALING™** Program, a comprehensive and transformative journey designed to empower women to achieve balance and harmony in all aspects of their lives. This program integrates the principles of quantum physics, holistic healing, nervous system regulation, growth, and self-awareness to address physical, emotional, mental, and spiritual well-being. Upon successful completion of the program, participants will be equipped with the knowledge, tools, and practices to continue their journey of self-discovery and holistic healing independently. If you are seeking a community of women who are on their healing journey, you may apply to work with me on our website www.storrie.co. I am a living proof that you can have both, a thriving business and health.

I am celebrating a 55-pound weight loss, making my health a priority as I am undergoing breast implant removal surgery.

There is a huge shift happening in the health and wellness industry. We are creating the **NEXT WAVE** of **PRACTITIONERS** who choose to become **WHOLISTIC WELLNESS COACHES™**. We are laser-focused on developing leaders in this industry. At the same time, we are witnessing Corporate America adding wellness programs for their employees. At STORRIE Wellness™, we are determined to bring Wholistic Wellness™ to Corporate America by providing many healing and energetic modalities to regulate the nervous system and support brain health. To learn more about our services, visit our website at www.storriewellness.com.

Through every pivot and shift in my business, I've had to face the realization that it's okay to change your mind. Your vision might change and develop into something totally different from what you had originally thought, and that is entirely OK. As you make decisions and enact changes over the course of your life, you will discover your lane as you go. That's the beautiful thing about life. We think that everything needs to happen on our timetable and the way we imagined. We create unnecessary suffering when things don't go the way we thought. Living your life thinking you have to control every situation will kill all your dreams and desires.

Remember, when you feel stuck, just **BREATHE**, commit to change so you can **HEAL**, and **SURRENDER**. Don't be so hard on yourself. Even if we have to rewrite our story over and over again, we have the freedom and opportunity to do so each and every day. As for my story, I know that we are just beginning to write the next chapter of combining all we offer at STORRIE Institute™ and STORRIE Wellness™ under one brand – STORRIE™, launching our brand new website www.storrie.co. If you're seeking a **COMMUNITY** that shares your passion for **Wholistic**

Wellness™, are taking purpose driven action towards their dream life, are creating their legacy with **Energetics of Entrepreneurship**™ in mind, all while making a positive **IMPACT** on the world, then you've found the perfect tribe: STORRIE™. There is so much more to come as we are continually building programs that serve people worldwide and will last for generations to come. In this chapter, I am choosing to rely on my breath to guide me, continue my healing journey as I prepare for my breast explant surgery, and simply surrender to the outcome.

I want you to rewrite your story and live your dream life. Place one hand on your belly, one hand on your heart. Close your eyes. Take a deep breath into your belly, take a deep breath into your heart, and exhale out. After each exhale, repeat after me.

I ask my intuition to take me to my destiny.
I ask the universe to surround me with mentors who will guide me.
I ask for everything that is not in alignment
with my highest path to go away.
I ask myself to forgive me for being so hard on myself.
I ask myself to forgive me for trying to be perfect.
I ask myself not to give up on the person I am becoming.
I ask my breath to guide me to my next step toward my dream life.

"Healing is not just a process; it's a quantum dance between our thoughts, emotions, and the universe, creating harmony within and around us. Awaken the healer in you." – Dr. Christine Manukyan

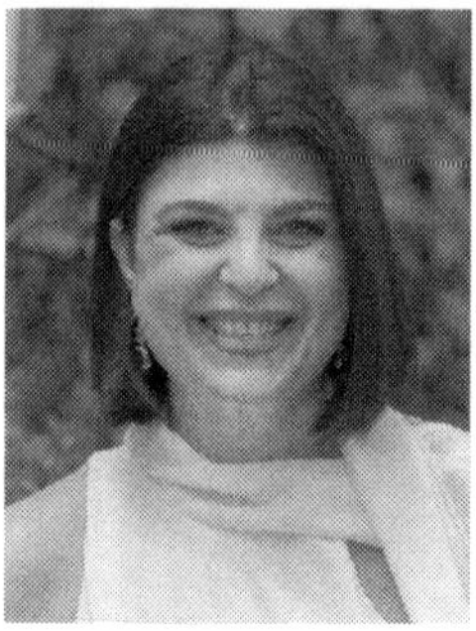

ABOUT DR. CHRISTINE MANUKYAN,
PHARMD, MS

Dr. Christine Manukyan is a pharmacist turned Corporate Wellness Strategist, Business Mentor, Wholistic Wellness Coach™, Certified Breathwork Practitioner, 4x bestselling author, speaker and top-ranked STORRIE™ Podcast host. As the Founder and CEO of two companies, STORRIE Institute™ and STORRIE Wellness™, she is pioneering the field of holistic health, leading the Wholistic Wellness Revolution™, and creating the new gold standard of care.

Prior to becoming an entrepreneur, she spent 13 years in Corporate America in various leadership roles. After experiencing her own health transformation with Functional Medicine, losing 100+ lbs and becoming a natural bodybuilding athlete and marathon runner, she found her true calling empowering others to reach their health goals without pharmaceuticals.

Dr. Christine holds several Board Certifications as a Clinical Hypnotherapist, Neuro-Linguistic Programing (NLP) Practitioner, Emotional Freedom Technique (EFT) Practitioner, Reiki Level 1 & 2 Practitioner, Time Techniques™ Practitioner, FIRES Coaching™ Practitioner and Life

& Success Coaching Practitioner. She is certified in Gene Testing (i.e. Nutrigenetics, Nutrigenomics and Pharmacogenomics), Sound Bowl Healing, Chakra Healing. Dr. Christine is a lifelong learner, completing courses from Harvard Medical School and Harvard Business School. She is currently enrolled in Quantum University for Doctorate in Holistic Health Program (class of 2024) and is in a process to become Certified NeuroSomatics Practitioner focusing on nervous system regulation and somatic healing.

She is a frequent speaker on Wholistic Wellness™, Energetics of Entrepreneurship™, Breathwork, Quantum Wholistic Healing™, creating thriving virtual wellness practice, founder and entrepreneur mindset, energy healing and nervous system regulation. She has spoken in front of audiences numbering 15,000+ and has been recognized globally for her entrepreneurial achievement and dedication. Her past publications and magazine features include FORBES, Yahoo, ABC, CBS, Entrepreneurs Herald, Disruptors, Authority Magazine, The News Universe, Daily Herald and BRAINZ Magazine.

Dr. Christine believes that everyone deserves a second chance to rewrite their story and become their ultimate best self.

www.storrie.co | drchristine@storrie.co | IG: @dr.christinemanukyan

Subscribe to The STORRIE™ Podcast

Join our private community on FB: Energetics of Entrepreneurship
www.facebook.com/groups/energeticsofentrepreneurship/

Join our private community on FB: Quantum Wholistic Healing
www.facebook.com/groups/quantumwholistichealing/

MY JOURNEY OF HOPE AND HEALING

By: Dr. Sarah Al Alam,
PHARMD, CSWWC

"You are most qualified to help the person you used to be."
– Ed Mylett

If you had a chance to rewrite your story, would you take the leap of faith and do it?

When I heard Ed Mylett say that quote, it changed my life. I knew somehow, someway, all the struggles and hardships that I had gone through would one day help someone just like me and I could be there for them in a way that I could empathize with them. Even though I didn't know how or what, I was determined to figure out a way to do that.

I was trained in the world of medicine and prescriptions and treating a problem after it arises. However, through my own personal journey, I have become passionate about the world of holistic health and healing; I will share why in my story to come. I would have to leave behind a world that was comfortable to be in and start my own journey into the world of the unknown.

Let me first introduce myself. My name is Dr. Sarah Al Alam. I am a wife, a mom of three, a sister, a daughter, a pharmacist, and so much more. I was born in Fall River, Massachusetts. I am a first-generation American. My family is from Lebanon. Although I was physically born here, I was raised the Lebanese way. Looking back, I am truly grateful for where I come from, but growing up I never really felt like I fit in anywhere. To me, I didn't fit in with the people who were born in Lebanon because I didn't think or speak the way they did. With the kids in my class, we didn't think the same way either, and the cultures were very different, from language to food to religion. I was baptized Orthodox but went to a Maronite Church because it was closer to where we lived. The majority of the kids in school were Roman Catholic. I remember in middle school lying about my background so I could fit in and be Irish or Portuguese like all the other kids in my class.

The way I was brought up was different from how the other kids were brought up. I wasn't allowed to have sleepovers, boys as friends, or even play sports if boys were on the team. I remember, I think it was in 5th grade, I was so excited that my mom had finally signed me up for the basketball team, but then once my parents realized there were boys on the team, they made me stop.

From a very young age, I remember I just wanted people to like me, to see me. I just wanted to fit into the world around me. Maybe this is one of the reasons I became a people pleaser? I did what I thought would make others happy as a way to feel like I fit in, like I belonged. It also didn't help that in our culture, everyone needs to know everyone's business – they need to know what you are doing, who you are with, and even what you are wearing. I felt like I was constantly being judged, which made me withdraw even more.

My mom was a stay-at-home mom. In the old Lebanese tradition, the husbands are the providers – they work and support the family while the mom stays home and takes care of the kids, cooks, cleans, etc. Once upon a time, I thought I wanted that too, but now after a lot of work on myself, I know I need more in my life. But that way of thinking has caused strain in my marriage.

It was not until recently that I started taking control over my life and not caring what other people thought or wanted. It was a scary step, and it still is scary, but I can't spend my life trying to please everyone else, because I know I will never truly be happy that way.

To add on top of trying to fit in and be liked, I was a chubby kid. Looking back, I am so grateful that my mom never called me fat or chubby, because I think it would have lowered my self-esteem more, but I remember her buying me "husky" clothes and telling me in a nice way to stop eating. Being chubby (in my eyes) did not help my case to try to fit in. And it didn't help that my two sisters were skinny, so I felt even more alone. In turn, I had very low self-esteem.

This turned into an eating disorder in middle school. I remember buying a pair of jeans that I really wanted, but they were too small for me. I was determined to lose the weight to fit into those jeans. Then, once I did that, people would like me and want to be my friend, or so I told myself.

I think my need to always be in control started at that moment. I lost the weight – mostly by starving myself because it was the only way I knew how – and fit into those jeans. I was proud of myself for maybe one day, but I had to lose more. I had to keep going. It was not enough. I ended up losing so much weight, my mom got worried, my period stopped coming, and I had to go to a nutritionist. I didn't care. It was the only thing that I could control, and I didn't know how to stop, so I just kept going.

Middle school was also around the time when I started having stomach issues. I think they started out because of anxiety because I hated middle school – everything about it, but those stomach issues followed me all the way to adulthood. So did the low esteem and never feeling like I was good enough. The stomach issues would be my door into a more holistic approach to healthy living.

The sad part was that losing weight didn't make me feel like I fit in any more than when I was chubby, and the same few amazing friends I had stayed with me no matter how I looked.

I share these stories because never feeling like I belonged and never feeling enough has affected me all my life. Those traumatic experiences growing up were not huge or super traumatic compared to what others have gone through, but I grew up feeling I was not good enough. And even to this day, it is something I struggle with.

I always waited for the outside validation to tell me I was good enough. I never went inward and told myself I was good enough. The way you talk and think about yourself means EVERYTHING. You need to be your first supporter, and everyone else will follow. I wish I knew that when I was younger.

I used to think being different was a bad thing, but today I know that being different is a way to stand out. I was always the type who wanted to be invisible in a crowd. If no one saw me, I wouldn't have to say anything, and then I would just blend in. Now I want my voice to be heard, and I want people to see me for who I really am. I want to be a support for others so they, too, don't have to feel alone. I am trying to be my own authentic self in the best way I can.

In my freshman year in college, I took a career finder test. Pharmacist was one of the answers. I was always good in the sciences, and I knew I wanted to do something in the healthcare field but not be in school for a million years. So, when I lost my grant for sophomore year (not grade-related) and there was an opening at Massachusetts College of Pharmacy and Health Sciences in Boston, I took it as a sign that it was the right choice for me, so I transferred out.

I hated pharmacy school. I feel like I missed out on the whole college experience. It felt like more of a graduate program than a time of self-discovery. I had one true friend there who was the best friend anyone could ask for. I think it was worse because freshman year I went to a liberal arts college, had the time of my life, then had no choice but to transfer out. Anyway, I did the best I could and tried to make the most out of the situation. I worked on weekends as an intern in the hospital, and the rest of the time I was studying. I really wanted to do a residency in ambulatory care because I thought that was the best way for me to make a difference and help people. Unfortunately, I didn't match with any residency program. The hospital I was working at had no openings at the time, and I just accepted a position in a retail setting. I told myself it would be a "for now" thing until I gained some experience and then I would move on.

My grandparents had a Lebanese bakery in Fall River, and I worked there in high school and college during breaks. I loved it because it was so busy, and I was good at it because I needed that fast-paced environment, otherwise, I would just get bored and restless. Retail was a whole different story.

I remember my first shift on my own. I failed miserably. It was just a four-hour shift, but I got the team so far behind. I could not check the prescriptions fast enough; everything was getting backed up. I cried on the way home. I told myself that was never going to happen again. I trained some more, then floated from store to store, then worked the overnight shift for a bit. I hated those. I still get PTSD thinking about them. I was a new graduate, didn't have much retail experience, and was put on overnights, where I was to work mostly by myself. Makes sense right? Eventually, I was placed at a consistent store and became a manager. I was so proud of myself to have made it to a pharmacy manager position. However, it came with a price. I lost so much sleep working as a manager. I was always nervous and on edge. I would come in early and stay late without getting paid. It was all a numbers game. It slowly became less and less about making a difference and more about meeting metrics and sales. It always came down to money.

When I got pregnant with my daughter, I wanted nothing to do with managing and being on call 24/7. I decided to take a step down from managing to being a staff pharmacist. In the 10 years I've been in retail, I've learned that I do well with a team. My technicians always knew that I had their back and I cared about them. They are probably the only reason why I have stayed in retail for so long. But, unfortunately, we are just a number to a big corporation. We are easily replaceable, and it doesn't matter how long you have been in the company. We work like slaves having to meet the demands of ridiculous metrics, like answering the phone in three rings. Honestly, there is no time for anything. I often felt like I was one person who was juggling so many tasks that made me feel overwhelmed and under constant pressure. It was not what I went to school for. I was also not aligned to what I was doing anymore.

When COVID hit, it changed everything. Talk about a toxic work environment. On top of filling prescriptions, we now had to give COVID vaccines, and some stores even had to do testing. We were not prepared for the amount of work given to us. We did not have the staffing for it. It was a dark time in the healthcare world. We were always days behind, we stopped answering the phones, patients were getting frustrated, and nothing was ready on time. It was too much. That is when I first heard the term "burnout." We never had the help we needed, we were constantly understaffed, and worst of all, I rarely felt appreciated in anything I did.

What started off as a "for now" job turned into a job of convenience. I ended up getting married, buying a house, and now have three beautiful children. As much as I knew retail was mentally destroying me, the schedule worked with my kids' schedule, and I was good at it. I was good at what I did, and I was scared to venture out and try something different because it was all that I knew.

Turning point:

In February of 2020 – the month before COVID hit – I knew I needed a change. I knew there had to be something better out there for me. This was not how I envisioned my life as a healthcare provider would be. I partnered up with a network marketing health and wellness company that my fellow pharmacist friend had also joined. I had no idea what network marketing was, but it opened the door to a whole new world for me, a world I didn't even know existed.

I was trained in the world of medicine and prescriptions, but to be completely honest, I was not aligned to what I was doing anymore.

When I learned I had to put myself out there for the business, I almost quit right then and there. You see, I am a Type-A perfectionist, and

I am also an introvert, so change or new situations does not come easy for me. However, I knew that if I didn't do anything to change my situation, then nothing would change, and I would stay stuck and depleted, and I didn't want that anymore. So I took a chance on myself and decided to give this health and wellness company a try. What did I have to lose?

I decided to do a 30-days-to-healthy-living reset, and I recruited my husband to do it with me. My friend, who was also a pharmacist, said it would help with my stomach issues. In my head, I didn't believe her since all my doctors, including Gastrointestinal doctors, I had already seen were unable to help. I honestly just did it to support my husband, who had been struggling with high cholesterol. Nothing he had tried had helped, and this was his last thing to try before the doctor was going to put him on medication. Even as a pharmacist I didn't want my husband on medication, because I knew it was going to be his easy way out to eat whatever he wanted, and that's not healthy either. The results of that total body reset changed my life. Would you believe just two weeks after doing this program, I no longer had stomach issues? I could for the first time in forever eat whatever I wanted, and I wasn't in excruciating pain. My husband, re-checked his blood work when he finished, and his cholesterol was for the first time since I knew him normal!

We are not taught about diet, nutrition, and sustainable healthy living in pharmacy school. We are taught about medications and disease states, but if you can help someone in a more holistic way, wouldn't that be better? If you could take simple steps to prevent something before it occurred, wouldn't that be better? I was slowly slipping away from the world of medication. I loved learning about nutrition, healing our bodies more naturally, and focusing on preventative care instead of just treating diseases as they come.

I heard this once and it just stuck: We don't have a healthcare system, we have a sick care system. I often speak with patients who are taking medications without knowing why their doctor prescribed them. That's because of the way the system is right now and how everything is all about money, no one has time for you anymore. I personally do not have time to talk to someone who comes to consultation or has a question on the phone. No one listens to what you are saying. It is easy to prescribe a pill for something and send the patient on their way. In a lot of situations, it's like putting a BAND-AID on the problem. You are not addressing the root cause, you are just covering it up with a prescription (BAND-AID). Do not get me wrong – there is a time and place for medications, but I just feel like these days it's easier to just prescribe someone a medication because it's the easy thing to do. But I think people forget that medications have side effects too.

With the pressures of work getting worse and worse, my kids at home were the ones paying the price. Because I was always in chaos and noise, when I got home I could not hear one more thing. When you have kids, that is not really an option. I didn't know how to handle and control my nervous system at home.

There is something else I need to add to make my story more complete. Everything I have mentioned so far has in some way shaped the course of my journey. It is regarding my son, George. Because I am strong in my faith I believe, although some days are not easy, that God does not give us anything we can't handle.

I was so excited to learn I was having a boy, especially coming from a Lebanese background. They love their boys. George is the biggest momma's boy and sweetest kid, but he has a hard time controlling his behaviors and emotions. His occupational therapist said he gets over-excited and has a hard time settling down.

George was a delayed speaker. I remember him using sign language to tell us what he wanted. And he was constantly whining. Always whining. Always. He would drive me nuts. We put him in early intervention for speech. His speech got better, but behavior issues were still there.

He would constantly be writing on our walls, spilling water on the floor, writing on beds and couches, and annoying his sisters. On his third birthday, he shoved a Q-tip in his ear and perforated his ear drum. We spent his birthday at Urgent Care.

I thought I was doing something wrong. It was literally like talking to a wall. Whether I would scream or try to stay calm, nothing seemed to work. He throws things when he gets mad, bangs on things, has tantrums, and breaks down when he doesn't get what he wants, or when he doesn't know how to respond to what he wants.

He gets overstimulated and over-excited easily, and is also sensitive to loud sounds, although that is slowly getting better.

I remember going to a Lebanese church party once. It was outside, and there was a Lebanese singer. I love doing things as a family, but they were not always that simple. We ordered our food – it was me, my husband, my two daughters, George, my parents, and aunts. Some cousins were there too. There were a lot of people, and it was loud. George started screaming and crying, saying it was too loud. He covered his ears with his hands, just screaming and crying. I tried to comfort him with little relief. I moved to the end of the tent toward the back of the tent and sat outside of it. Poor thing was screaming. All the other kids and parents seemed to be having fun. I felt alone. I felt like no one understood me. Was I doing something wrong? As hard as I tried I could not comfort him.

This wasn't the only time this happened. It also happened at the parade, a baptism, and a Halloween event. These are the ones I could remember.

I can't tell you how many times I cried. A *lot.* I cried that I didn't think I was a good mom because I didn't know what to do. I didn't know how to help him. I knew he couldn't control his emotions, but I was in a state where neither could I. Those feelings that I had felt in middle school of feeling alone, unseen, and misunderstood were coming back, and I hated it and it only added to my anxiety.

Everyone kept telling me he was a typical Lebanese boy, and you know what, maybe they were right, or maybe not. All I knew was I was so drained from life mentally that I couldn't emotionally handle it.

Between being overwhelmed and stressed at work and coming home to the same environment, I was slowly breaking down inside.

It didn't help that my husband and I have very different parenting beliefs, and this caused a strain on our relationship. We never seemed to agree on anything. I was focusing so much attention on George that my other kids were not getting the attention they needed or deserved.

With all the pressures at work and home and kids and marriage, I think I just lost it. I lost myself. I didn't know who I was anymore or what my purpose was in life anymore. Yes, I am a mother, but I knew something deep down inside was missing.

I was on this hamster wheel and couldn't stop spinning.

I knew there had to be a better way.

I spent so long self-diagnosing George and trying to come up with a diagnosis so I could treat him, but that's exactly the problem with our healthcare system.

Unless you have a diagnosis, no one knows how to treat you or give you medicine.

One day I realized I didn't care if he had a diagnosis or not. I was talking with my life coach and a light bulb went off.

I realized that in order to help calm Gerogi's nervous system, I had to help myself first. I knew my anxieties and constant stress were rubbing off not only on Georgi but on the other kids as well. I could feel it, but I just didn't know what to do or how to handle it.

Because I was surrounded with so much noise and chaos all the time, I was constantly overstimulated. To be honest, given the world we live in now, it's easy to be overstimulated.

I had to learn how to protect my energy and protect my peace, because inside I felt like a volcano was about to explode all the time. I was always nervous and always stressed, and I was tired of feeling that way. I wanted to be one big happy family, but I felt like we were falling apart.

The day I heard Ed Mylett speak in person was the day that changed my life. "You are most qualified to help the person you used to be."

With all the struggles I went through from feeling burnout in my career, my health, Georgi, my kids, my family, my marriage, maybe I could turn it around and help someone like me. I know God has a plan for me, I just had to have faith that it would all work out in the end. I want to turn my pain into purpose.

I know as parents we are supposed to teach our children. George has taught me so much about myself and what I need to feel better. In trying to soothe and calm George, I have learned so much about calming my own nervous system. For example, George is very affectionate and loves hugs and cuddles. Guess what? You know what helps calm me down? A gentle touch, a warm hug, someone telling me everything is going to be OK. I wanted to be seen, heard, and understood, and so did he in his own way.

It's funny how we both needed the same thing. In that journey to self-discovery, I fell in love with the world of healing and holistic medicine. I could have easily gotten on medication to help me but chose not to. I wanted to heal myself from the inside. And I want the same for George too.

I started off by adapting a healthier lifestyle for me and my family. I stopped eating and buying junk food and household products and started investing in cleaner non-toxic everyday household products.

Did you know that certain artificial dyes or colors in the food industry today like the red 40 or yellow 6 can make some children's behavior worse?

Well, we cut those out.

I have also done other things to help me heal:

- Hired mentor/life
- Hired a personal trainer to help me get physically and mentally stronger
- Limited social media
- Surrounded myself with people who were going to lift me up and inspire me
- Started doing breathwork/meditation
- Journaling
- Understanding my human design
- Learning how to sit still in the chaos

- A community for me is huge–just being around people who understand you makes all the difference
- Therapy
- SLOW DOWN
- Getting outside

For Georgi:

- Nutrition
- Supplementation
- A minimum of 30 minutes outside time a day
- Sleep – this one is super-important, especially for kids who are constantly going
- Chiropractor
- Positive reinforcement
- Timers
- Limiting electronics

For the high-achieving mom in healthcare who on the outside seems to have everything together but on the inside you are falling apart … I see you, I feel you, I understand you. I want you to know you are not alone.

Are your negative emotions and anxieties transferring to your kids and now you are all in a state of dysregulation and chaos?

Or maybe you just need someone who understands you? Are you struggling with a difficult child and just need some tools and strategies to make your day a little calmer?

If you are like me, I just want you to know you are not alone.

I have done a lot to help myself heal and be a better person. I am slowly learning to surrender to the things I cannot control.

Please do not get the wrong idea. I still have my struggles and insecurities that I am working through. I am far from perfect, but I am learning every day how I can be a better person, not only for myself but for my family too.

Here is my vision: To help and support moms like me.

I know how important one-on-one coaching is where we focus on you, Healing you. I promise I will listen to what you need and will support you in any way I can. I also know how important a community aspect is. That is why I plan to have both. It's nice to know you are not the only one dealing with certain situations and that you are not alone.

I'm also realizing that as much as I feel like I need to know everything, I know that is not possible. So, I can bring in the experts to help – things I wish I had – like a children's psychologist, couples therapist, breathwork session, life coach, nutritionist, energy healing, meditation, and so on.

I felt alone for a large part of my life, even though I physically was not alone, but I felt no one understood me. I don't want anyone to feel that.

Everyone deserves to feel loved, heard, and seen.

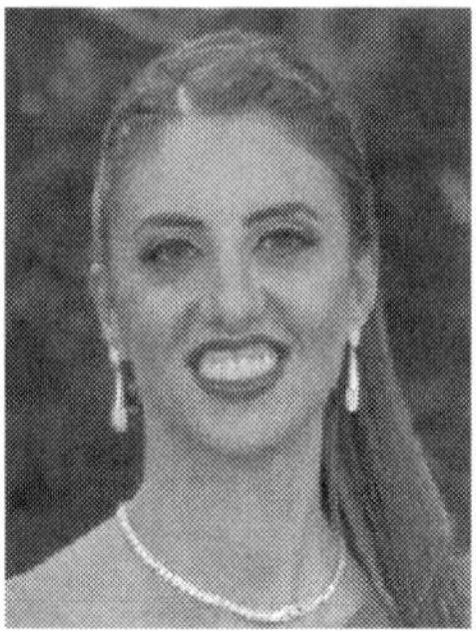

ABOUT DR. SARAH AL ALAM,

PHARMD, CSWWC

Dr. Sarah Al Alam brings a unique blend of influences as a first-generation American with a Lebanese heritage. A licensed Pharmacist, who is also on a transformative journey to become a Certified STORRIE Wholistic Wellness Coach™ (CSWWC) through the renowned STORRIE Institute™.

With over a decade of experience, Dr. Sarah Al Alam's journey started with versatility and evolved into a deep passion for health and wellness during a personal health journey with her husband.

She believes healing goes beyond medication. It involves understanding our bodies, making lifestyle changes, and embracing practices like breathwork.

As a mother of three, she's committed to helping others find their healing paths. Her youngest son's unique nervous system journey has taught her about managing stress and finding balance.

Dr. Sarah humbly admits she doesn't have all the answers, but she's committed to growth—for herself and others.

sarahalalam88@gmail.com | LI: @sarahalalampharmd |
IG: @sarahkristen1013

THE POWER OF BEING YOU: LIVING A REAL, RAW, AND AUTHENTIC LIFE OUT LOUD WITH CHRONIC ILLNESS

By: Sarah Brooke Berg,
BAWS, BCC, LPN, CHt, CRP, CSWWC

"At the end of the day, the best thing you can do is live. Make the memories, eat the damn food, and be present in your life. Stop chasing the newest health fad and just listen to your body and treat her like you love her. That's the secret to true health."

– Sarah Brooke Berg

Every day there is someone out there who is walking around in pain not even realizing how abnormal that is. Maybe that is you right now. Back pain? Foot pain? PMS? I know it was me for the longest time. See, my story starts from when I was a baby – the sickness, hospital visits, my parents not knowing any better and thinking that the doctor's word was the end-all and be-all. But before we get into that, it's important for you to know the absolute magic that can exist within the holistic health world.

If you are anything like me, that world might feel very confusing. When I first started studying holistic health and what it meant, I couldn't understand it at all. Every person who talked about it seemed to have conflicting information. For example, one person would say garlic is so great for you, and anyone with thyroid conditions should be using it, only for the next person to say garlic is a nightshade, and people with thyroid conditions should avoid it completely. This was everywhere, and it left me more confused than anything. Stay away from inflammatory oils, don't eat processed foods, no sugar, no caffeine, only alkaline water … I started to get confused about what I *could* eat.

I became obsessive, very quickly. I was checking the labels of every food, spending more money than I had on groceries, I really didn't have at the time, but I didn't care – I was desperate for a change. I also had a false sense of what true holistic health was, thinking if I did this and stuck to it, I would be skinny and, well, that was a whole other battle to conquer. It took me years, specifically the pandemic, to realize how absolutely messed up my idea of holistic wellness truly was. At this point I had been a nurse for about six years and was in school for Ayurveda wellness and Integrative Medicine. I understood a lot about the Western medicine world, and my eyes were starting to open to what true holistic health was.

Ayurveda is an ancient medical system that is over 5000 years old. It is the science of life and knowledge. Ayurveda believes that imbalances and disease occur in a person's physiology when stress and inflammation are present. Ayurveda encourages many different healing modalities to help a person live a fulfilling life, full of health and wellness instead of disease, but when disease is present, there are plenty of interventions that will help a person regain balance. This was the type of holistic health I could get behind, the kind of health advice that is based on a person rather than a protocol that we just give to everyone and their brother.

When we do that, we miss the human experience, we miss the person we are helping. We are not all the same, and that is where Western medicine messes up as well. We need to treat the individual rather than the disease, understanding what they have access to. We need to treat the disease with a root approach rather than a blanket solution. This was something I craved. This was something I needed for myself and what I loved learning to further help clients. Getting to the root cause meant understanding why someone had high blood pressure rather than just giving them a medication for high blood pressure, then dealing with the side effects of said medication. If we slow down, maybe we can figure out that this person is dealing with a stressful environment and needs nervous system support rather than be on medication for the rest of their lives. This was whole-body health, this was true holistic health, and this was something I knew so many needed.

My curiosity only peaked from there, and as I started my clinicals for my bachelor's degree, I learned how to help my clients on such a deeper level. I knew I couldn't wait to apply this to my clients and help them with their digestion, reproductive issues, inflammation, fatigue, brain fog, respiratory issues, and hormone health. Helping them get to the root cause of the issue rather than just a medicine that helps them for a month until the side effects of the medicine outweigh the benefits. Being an Ayurveda Holistic Health Practitioner has changed my life, and that is just a small part of why I knew this was for me. Being able to provide care to my family and friends, and helping my clients, has been so rewarding: seeing how they are finally relieved from their high blood pressure and cholesterol; seeing how they are finally experiencing normal digestion, and understanding the importance of stress relief with meditation and yoga; showing plus-size women that you don't need to lose weight to become a healthier you, but rather how to implement certain modalities that lead to true health, and sometimes through that weight comes off naturally; showing my patients that true health comes from loving the body they are in and treating it right, leaving diet culture and what society makes us feel is "healthy" and turning inward and listening to the body … that's what being a holistic practitioner means to me.

As I continued to help patients, I still realized there was a gap, a mindset that seemed to be a huge struggle, and I wondered how I could help that. That is when a coaching program fell into my lap, and I realized if I wanted to give my clients the results they wanted and give them true health, then I needed to help them with their mindset as well. Working with the subconscious mind as a board-certified life coach helped me help them on a deeper level. See, change can happen on the surface level, but how many times have you tried something and it didn't stick? You wanted it so badly and were confused as to why you couldn't make it work. It is because the change needs to happen on the subconscious level, the level that makes up 99 percent of your decision-making, and to do that, you need to be using the right language.

The other part I found lacking was the energy, and when I became a life coach, I learned very quickly how to incorporate that for my clients. Using modalities like hypnotherapy, Reiki, timeline techniques, parts integration, and fire methods helped me facilitate deep inner healing, release work, and so much more. This created more room for clients to focus on the healing of their body and drop out of their mind, meaning instead of living in your head where all the noise is, I guide you on how to drop into your body and listen there. This is truly a topic I can talk about forever, because energy work is just as important as holistic health work, if not more important! It's going to be very difficult to heal your leaky gut if you still have deep feelings of hurt, grief, anger, etc., present in your system. You must process these to make room for true health, and if you don't, it will only manifest into disease in your organs, tissues, etc. This work is potent, and I wanted to provide it so my patients had one place where they could go, instead of having to refer them out and build that trust with someone else, because it is so difficult to do and for me I wouldn't be able to or at least it would take a long time to open up about stuff like this, as in traumas the body and mind has stored or limiting beliefs that are present. This is what I believe a true holistic health practice should look like for patients. Yes, the lab work is important, and yes, understanding your digestion and what food does to your body is important, but the energy work is just as important, and processing your emotions is just as important. I get it, it may not be sexy to cry it out, to take a minute to breathe, to regulate your nervous system, but if you don't, I can promise you, you are wasting your time.

There have been multiple times in my life where Western medicine has failed me. When I was a baby, I was sick all the time, spent a lot of time in hospitals in an asthma tent, and had chronic ear infections and chronic strep throat, which meant chronic use of antibiotics and never building my good gut bacteria back up because the science wasn't there at the time (or at least wasn't widely known – Ayurveda literature talks about this). If you know anything about holistic health, you know a lot of disease starts in the gut, and with mine weak from chronic antibiotic use, you can imagine how this story is going to go.

As I grew up I struggled with the weirdest skin issues and was on constant steroids for them, tonsilitis was flaring up every time I turned around, and eventually, my tonsils were removed. Lab work was done, and little did we know (because it was never shared with us), I was showing signs of hyperthyroidism. Two years later, my life changed forever. I woke up with a goiter around my neck. If you don't know what that is, much like my mother and I didn't, it looks like you swallowed a tire. A quick trip to the ER established that I had something called Graves' disease, an autoimmune condition that can be absolutely life-threatening. With my thyroid levels the way they were, I was quickly sent to a specialist who confirmed it, and put me on thyroid and heart medications. I was 12, and although hospitals didn't scare me because I was used to them (I was rather fascinated with them), I was absolutely scared of this. The seriousness behind everyone's faces is what scared me. I could feel the tenseness of the situation, and when the medication wasn't working, it only got worse. I don't remember much of this. That's the thing about the body – it has a beautiful mechanism of protection. Forget everything so it doesn't hurt, and that's exactly what my mind did.

Everything is fuzzy, but the few pieces I do remember, I understand why my brain said, "Nope we aren't remembering this." Protection. What I do remember is going into a room that looked like a lab, and having to drink something that tasted like gross water. It was radioactive, and it basically "nuked" my thyroid. I had to stay away from friends and family for a few days and use a separate restroom because I was radioactive. All of this was while someone who I considered to be a father figure passed away, and I couldn't go to the funeral, because I was radioactive. Talk about trauma.

After the procedure, there was no further follow-up with the endocrine pediatric doctors, which would turn out to be one of the biggest mistakes that would affect my life forever. My mother had no idea, and I know to this day that is the one thing she would take back in a heartbeat. Everything since that moment has changed, and I would never be the same. The thing is, my mother was a single parent most of the time. The father who adopted me didn't believe I had anything wrong with me and would oftentimes poke at me, saying I was a hypochondriac, so my mother did a lot of parenting alone. When you go to a specialist who you assume knows best, you trust them, especially because 20 years ago, what a doctor said was gold. There was no reason not to trust them. Fast forward four years. I am in my senior year of high school, and I have a moon face and have gained 75 pounds out of nowhere. I'm super active, I eat decent meals, I am in cheerleading, I work out, my job has me on my feet for over eight hours a day, and the weight keeps coming on no matter what I do. Trust me … I do everything to stop it, including developing an eating disorder.

I'm not alone when I say that I was searching high and low for answers, along with my mom, who noticed a massive change in me, and that's when we stumbled onto my first holistic doctor. I had to apply to be in her practice. I wrote an essay and shared a picture of my weight gain with her because for me, that was the only thing that mattered, and I was accepted into her practice. At first, things were wonderful. I finally felt a sense of relief, and even though I was taking about 15 different supplements and medications and my diet was severely restricted because of my "food allergies," I was finally seeing the weight come off. She diagnosed me with post-ablative Hashimoto's disease, meaning the small part of my thyroid that was left from the nuking was creating antibodies to attack itself. We didn't even know that was possible.

I found out that the doctors should have followed up with me. Four years of having my thyroid attack itself left my body in flight-or-fight mode, my adrenals were toast, my body was exhausted, and emotionally, I was not in a good place, but no one knew that part. Sometimes I wish the "me now" could go back in time, and shake the 17-year-old I was, and tell her, "He's not worth it, focus on you because this is the only body you will get." Fast forward a few months, and I was in college, living in a dorm, going to nursing school, and still had my high school boyfriend. He had been cheating on me and ignoring me, which led to me spiraling quickly, not focusing on myself and the major medications and diet restrictions I was supposed to be following, and then adding alcohol into the mix because I was heartbroken and in a sorority, and well I think you could guess what happened from there. A very sick, sick Sarah, who flunked nursing school, ended up finding out my boyfriend of four years had been cheating on me from a phone call from him on February 14th and, well, the rest is history.

I had to tell my family what happened, went home, enrolled in the community college right away, and started again, with a 45-minute commute to school and my health issues still a major problem. I failed nursing school AGAIN, thanks to adrenal stress fatigue and always being sick. This time I took a semester off and started to heal, and really tried to follow what I needed, but I was still heartbroken and had no idea how to process. This time in my life was probably the most damaging, and it's still something that at 30 years old I am processing and forgiving. One day, I will share this story but for now, know that I finally passed nursing school, married my love, and followed him around the U.S. as he is in active duty military.

That wasn't the end of my health issues though. As a newlywed, I couldn't figure out why I had so many issues with exhaustion that led to me not wanting intimacy. When I went to the military doctor, she said, "Well it makes sense, you are away from your family, you are a new nurse, and newly married – give yourself a break." I appreciated that feedback back then and took her word, but now I realize that my doctor wasn't a therapist, and she should have done a proper work-up rather than giving me life advice. Maybe then she would have found that I actually had endometriosis, PCOS (polycystic ovarian syndrome), and my IUD was misplaced. Instead, I waited about three years with worsening symptoms before I got the answers I needed. I wish this was the end of my health issues, but sadly, that was far from the case. I could write a whole book on this alone, and you probably wouldn't be able to wrap your mind around how my story goes, then again that's probably not true, and I am less alone than I think I am. Let me share what has stood out the most. I went to the foot doctor, because one of the lovely facts about thyroid conditions is that it's literally connected to your feet. I had been dealing with plantar fasciitis since I was 13, and was now 22 and working as a nurse.

At this point I had been in a healthcare career for six years, which means being on your feet ... A LOT! This particular encounter with the foot doctor left me defeated, as he attributed all of my foot issues to my weight, not knowing that I had been suffering from an eating disorder, over-exercising, under-eating, and he stated my foot issues were from my "belly." Specifically, he called it a wheat belly, yet did not ask about my diet, which at that time I had been restricting for a while: no gluten, no dairy, and checking every label excessively. I left that appointment feeling disgusted with myself, which led to more excessive measures. This wasn't the only instance a doctor has said fat-phobic comments to me, although, at the foot doctor visit, I wasn't fat at all.

Months after my second miscarriage, a doctor told me I had excess estrogen because of my fluffy tummy. She then documented in my medical chart that we would not be a good fit, because I told her that there was no actual science to back her diagnosis up and that I would like an actual medical work-up rather than her advice. One time I had a provider tell me it was absolutely safe to eat 500 calories a day and work out for more than an hour a day when I was working 12-hour shifts. Luckily I knew how unsafe that was and I didn't listen, but I can only think of the ones who did listen and are probably walking around with a wrecked metabolism and hormones that need a lot of repair.

After searching for answers for years, I finally stumbled upon a Functional Medicine dietician, and my life really changed. I finally had the correct lab testing ordered, and for once in my life, I received answers and support. We discovered I had parasites, *Helicobacter pylori*, heavy metal toxicity, and mold toxicity, and we immediately got to work healing, which has taken years of work. I saw some progress, then began to hit a standstill, and after years of research and learning, I knew deep down it because I needed to address my burnt-out nervous system which was still operating from a flight-or-fight mode. I still have a long way to go, and I have realized so much along the way, my biggest takeaway being if your nervous system isn't regulated, it's going to take a long time to heal. You can't outrun your trauma. It gets stuck in your muscles and tissues, and until you take the time to address that, you will only heal on the surface level. Process the hand you have been given, the pain, the hurt, the trauma, and then you can focus on the rest and finally feel free.

During these health issues I faced, I was heavy in an MLM (multi-level marketing), which I now know to be more of a cult. At the time, I thought I was doing amazing things, helping women lose weight and getting paid to do so, but something in 2020 flipped, and all of a sudden the language and verbiage I would use made me feel some type of way, like gross and judged, and I slowly stepped away. I started to look at the other side of things and the actual science behind dieting and diet culture. I was immediately shocked. I thought I had been on a journey of self-love through weight loss, but I could never figure out why enough wasn't actually enough. I never truly liked what I saw in the mirror, and my confidence was so surface-level. I really started to explore what this meant and looked like. I started eating some of my "off limits" food, I started to touch my body, and I explored what mirror work was. I was more gentle, kind, and eventually loving to my body. It was then I knew

I wanted to share this with more women. I wanted to reverse the damage I had done, and most importantly, I wanted to share what I had learned. So, I created a three-step coaching program, launched beta testing, and started confidence coaching. It was during this time I had hired my first business coach. She really showed me the ropes on what to do, and it was so simple after this. I had this deep faith within myself that I could help and that everyone would want to learn how to be confident. Before you knew it, I had several clients lined up and purchasing sessions and packages. They had amazing results, but it didn't feel like enough. It felt very surface-level.

During all of this, I was still researching confidence coaching, plus-size lifestyle, and diet culture, and that is when I found a coach whose style, confidence, and literally everything about her I adored. I followed her on Instagram, and absorbed all of her content. It was then that she started posting about something called the Quantum Ripple Effect (QRE) Institute, a life-coaching program that certifies students in about seven different healing modalities. I was interested and began talking to my husband about it, but was really sold when she mentioned, "Are you a coach who gives talk advice?" My immediate thought was fuck, that's me.

When she went on to talk about how this is only creating surface-level change, something I had already been noticing, and how NLP, one of the modalities they teach inside of QRE is much deeper than that and creates change on the subconscious level which in return creates lasting change, lasts I knew then I was sold and would do anything to be a part of this institute. I was already in school at this time for a bachelor's degree in Ayurveda Wellness and Integrative Medicine, but I knew I could do anything I put my mind to, and I did.

I hired her as my life coach to help my own healing journey, and she doubled as my business coach as well. I immediately started sharing about this and how I couldn't wait to incorporate it all. Soon after I was certified, I created more programs about self-love and confidence and incorporated Ayurveda as well. Helping women on their self-love journeys was my pride and joy. I loved seeing them bloom, their confidence grow, and finally getting out of their own way and living the life they deserved. After I graduated with my bachelor's degree, I started working at a local apothecary and hosting events, teaching Ayurveda, and helping women process stuck emotions. This has been my dream job, and although I still work as a nurse every now and then, I know I am exactly where I want to be. Soon I'll be master-certified, meaning I have extensive knowledge of the subconscious mind and how to help on a deeper level.

These days you can find me doing exactly that: helping women on a deep level; helping them heal their nervous system through somatic healing; helping them heal ailments they struggle with like digestion, metabolism, hormones, allergies, reproductive health, and any other health concerns that come up; and getting to do this through lab work, using my certifications, and also using Ayurveda to help support. This work is a do-with-the process, so although I am helping facilitate the healing and knowledge, I can do it for you, you have to be an active participant in your own journey. I like to explain it like this: We are in a car together, you are in the driver's seat, and I am like your GPS. I simply guide you to where you should go to reach your destination, but maybe along the way you want to take a detour or a different route. My role as your GPS is to simply reroute and find the next option. I'm always here to guide, support, and help, but at the end of the day, you are in the driver's seat, and ultimately you make the decision, which is always the right decision because you know your body best. At the end of the day, the women I work with are getting massive support in all areas of life in one place, which has massive ripples in their life and builds a bond and trust to really heal.

When I am not helping clients, you can find me on TikTok, Instagram, my website, YouTube, or Facebook. I love sharing my life like an open book and having so many certifications, licenses, and degrees. I am always teaching and sharing, and being married to the military keeps my life pretty entertaining. For the longest time, I struggled with feeling like I had to be a certain way as a nurse or even as an Ayurvedic Practitioner and Life Coach, but I know now (after receiving my own coaching) that people feel connected with me because I am real and raw and share it like it is. There is no holding back in my life, and I will always keep it that way. What you see, my personality is exactly what it is. My whole life I just wanted to be normal. Now, in my 30s, I crave to be wild, in love with life, the weird one, the one who is known to be eclectic, a hippie, my bubbly self, anything but normal. Helping women understand that true health has no look, true confidence has no bounds, and self-love can exist in the body you are in, is my calling. Being a professional can look like me showing up exactly how I am, dancing around in a bikini on the internet in my fat body, and I wonder if more people saw and believed this, how different the world would be, how, just maybe, we can change societal norms. If I have to leave you with anything, it is, be YOU. There is power in being yourself. There is power in your story, and your life, and being your authentic self even in your healing journey will lead you to the road of self-love and will bring safety to your body. I write this as I am experiencing this in my own journey. Having to sit down and type this chapter in a time in my life where everything just feels dull and mute. A time in my life where my whole world was flipped upside down, in the middle of a military move, finding out my husband was deploying soon, we would be traveling and living in hotels for months on end, and right before we leave getting the call that my father died very traumatically just days before I was going to see him. I can tell you the grief and regret has flipped my world upside down, very unexpectedly, but I share this with you because I am living proof of what I have shared in this chapter. Allow the breakdowns to come through and be breakthroughs, allow yourself to heal, take care of your body and nervous system, and see how the energetics can change your life. I believe in you, just like I have believed in myself, to show up, and write this, even when there were days I didn't know if it even mattered. Choose YOU, everyday.

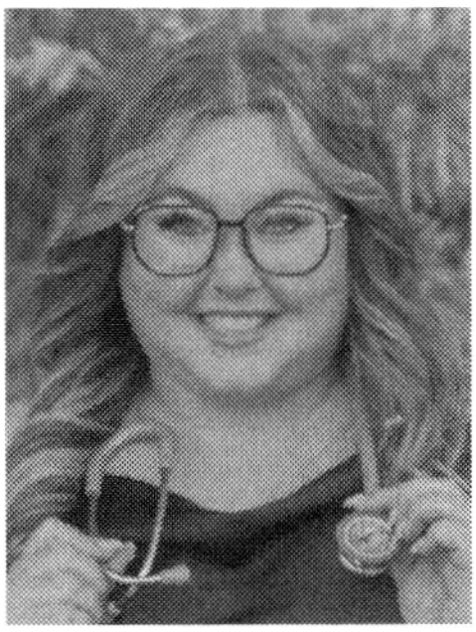

ABOUT SARAH BROOKE BERG,

BAWS, BCC, LPN, CHT, CRP, CSWWC

Sarah Brooke Berg is a Board Certified Life Coach, Ayurveda Practitioner, and Licensed Practical Nurse who started in the western medicine world but realized very quickly that there was a missing piece of the puzzle when serving her patients and went on a journey to figure out what that was. She is also in the process of becoming a Certified STORRIE Wholistic Wellness Coach™ (CSWWC) from STORRIE Institute™.

After going on her own journey in the holistic health world she quickly realized how important both worlds are and how combined, could really serve so many. Being her patient's biggest advocate and helping them bridge the gap between mental and physical health in both worlds has quickly become her passion. Sarah has now started her own business and practice, helps plus-size women fall in love with their bodies and gain the confidence they deserve, is becoming a Master Practitioner, and has helped over 200 people with health, true wellness, and finally live the peaceful life they deserve.

Sarah has been a nurse for almost 10 years and has worked in the healthcare field for over 14. Sarah has a bachelor's degree in Ayurveda wellness and Integrative Medicine, & has been a board-certified life coach for over 2 years. Sarah has a passion for both being a professional and living a real, raw, and free-spirited life and has learned that you can have your cake and eat it too by being a multifaceted woman.

Sarah enjoys spending time with her family, playing with her golden retriever Mia, and as a military spouse soaks up every moment with her husband. You can find her walking the beaches on Whidbey Island, at the local farmers market finding goodies, or at her favorite coffee shop working on her next project.

At Sarah Brooke Berg Co. you can expect an individualized approach to your health and wellness! Sarah specializes in plus size, self-love, body image, and confidence coaching, along with Ayurveda and functional medicine for every body type. The minute you walk into a session Sarah is using a trauma-informed approach and coaching to help you start to feel your best while being comfortable and in a safe environment.

Sarah uses 7 different healing modalities to help you see results in your life on a subconscious level, the area of the brain that makes up 99% of your decision-making, thus leading to lasting results and real change. Sarah also offers wellness consults that focus on you as an individual, paying focus to lifestyle, herbs, and aromatherapy to help prevent disease and leading you to live healthier and happier.

www.sarahbrookeberg.com | deeplyrootedayurveda@gmail.com |
IG: @sarahbrookebergco

CHARTING A NEW COURSE

By: Roger Benedetti,
RPH, BPHARM

*"If you do not change direction,
you may end up where you are heading."*
– Lao Tzu

It was a dark and stormy night …

Unlike the clichéd openings of fictional tales, this narrative was real. The elements of that evening dramatically set the stage, for this was no ordinary tale. Instead, it is a chronicle of my life's journey, an evolutionary story of a professional paradigm shift intertwined with my personal health transformation.

It began during a typical Florida summer evening thunderstorm when my wife, Cathy, and I arrived at her parents' home for a surprise visit. The purpose of our trip was to see for ourselves what was genuinely happening, because we suspected that her parents were only giving us incomplete information. "Everything is fine" is what they said on the phone. What we found broke our hearts. Her dad could not walk to the end of the driveway to pick up the newspaper without stopping to gasp for breath. Her mom was confused and disoriented. They were both overwhelmed with medical appointments, and fell short of maintaining their health and well-being despite their best efforts.

As a pharmacist, one area that was extra troublesome to me was the disarray of their medications and the number of vials that needed shoeboxes for storage. Although all were filled accurately by my colleagues, the medicines were not being taken correctly due to poor compliance, missed doses, and duplicate drugs that included both brands and generics of the same drugs. It was the definition of and an exemplification of polypharmacy at its worst.

I instinctively took immediate action, drawing upon my foundation in problem-solving skills and aptitude for systems thinking. I took the necessary steps to address the issue, established a comprehensive medication management system, coordinated with a new provider, and ensured I would have remote access for efficient medication management.

We knew we could not continue providing the needed care in person, and would have to return to our home and jobs in New Jersey. We sought help for improving their health and enabling them to remain independent at home. We enlisted service from a home care agency, alongside a registered nurse care manager, precisely the help needed for all involved. Knowing that her parents were being cared for enabled us to return home with peace of mind.

From a dark and stormy night emerged a beacon of light. The experience and challenges I encountered during this particular trip, which involved providing direct patient care outside the traditional pharmacy setting, sparked an unexpected response within me. I felt a strong urge to venture from behind the confines of the pharmacy counter and make an impact in a different environment in clients' homes, where medication adherence issues occur. Consequently, after enjoying a successful 25-year career, predominantly as a pharmacy manager in a major national retail pharmacy, I boldly decided to depart from the corporate world and embark on an entrepreneurial journey.

This resolve led to the founding and operation of a home care agency where I could leverage my background. The specific insights gained over the years from both being in the caregiver role from a distance and being a medical provider are unique within the home care industry. As a result, our company became established as a valuable resource and service provider of home care specifically tailored to the needs of seniors in the community.

Our new home care company received a request for a consultation from a concerned daughter. The story she shared began with her arrival at her mother's home late one evening after a long drive in the pouring rain. Sitting outside on the porch was her mother, alongside her packed suitcase. When the daughter asked her mother why, her mom said that she had to leave before the homeowners got home and found her there. After a struggle and still unable to convince her mother that it was her own home, the daughter got her to return inside. But the surprises were not over. She found so much more, from the old-fashioned coffee pot on the stove that was still burning with all the water boiled away, to the shower that was still running into a full bathtub. At this point, the daughter recognized it was time to get help for her mother, as she could no longer be safe alone in the home.

What stood out about this case was what happened during the admission, when the daughter mentioned that her mother recently began taking an antidepressant medication. This class of drug is known to have the potential to cause dementia-like symptoms. Based on my suggestion, the prescriber agreed to discontinue the medication. As if it was a miracle, her dementia improved, so much that the family felt they had their mom back again.

Seeing this change firsthand marked my initial encounter with the positive outcomes of reducing medication use. Previously, our Home Care company's focus revolved around telling our origin story and differentiating factor as a pharmacist-led organization, emphasizing the importance of safe, accurate, and efficient medication usage. Compliance held the utmost significance, and implementing medication reconciliation during transitions of care (admission, transfer, and discharge) proved to be the most effective strategy in preventing discrepancies and adverse drug events.

In a significant professional milestone, I witnessed a new treatment approach: Instead of prescribing medications, I saw the effectiveness of removing them. This process, known as deprescribing, involves the supervised reduction or cessation of medicines that may be causing harm or are no longer beneficial. Deprescribing is crucial in optimizing medication use, managing chronic conditions, minimizing adverse effects, and enhancing overall outcomes, particularly among older or sicker individuals. Unfortunately, the demand for this service has been relatively low, as home care typically falls within the conventional medicine continuum.

And so it was from another tale, also commencing with a dark and stormy night, that my curiosity was ignited and a new pathway in my professional and personal journey was illuminated, guiding me toward uncharted territories to navigate.

As I witnessed patients with chronic conditions not improving and aging prematurely, I started recognizing the constraints of the traditional approach in healthcare. Despite conventional practitioners recommending lifestyle changes, patients often struggle to adhere, and opt for medications instead, highlighting a system prioritizing pharmaceuticals, fostering the belief that medicine is preferable, a "pill for every ill." Consequently, due to passive care within the established system and a lack of active engagement in lifestyle modifications, patients fail to address the underlying causes and attain genuine healing.

Through my experiences, specifically in the field of home care, I discovered interesting patterns in the intricate relationship between medication, health, and the needs of our clients. A correlation existed between the number of medications a client took and their overall well-being. I found that the more drugs a person takes, the poorer their health, necessitating an earlier intervention in the form of in-home care assistance needed.

I noticed that our younger clients – those in their 50s and 60s – who took multiple medications often were in poor overall health. These individuals had various other health conditions, and their need for in-home care stemmed mainly from physical needs. On the other hand, I observed that among our older clients – those in their 80s or 90s – most were on few medications, were generally fitter, and required in-home care primarily due to the challenges faced at their advanced age.

As the basis for our care plan, I became deeply familiar with the term "activities of daily living" (ADL), a checklist used to assess the health and functionality of elderly people. The list includes basic tasks such as preparing a meal for oneself, walking without assistance, bathing, grooming, using a phone, going to the grocery store, handling personal finances, managing medications, and so on.

Working within senior care, I saw the vast differences in the longevity of our clients and learned about the components of lifespan and healthspan. Conventional medicine primarily focuses on lifespan and almost entirely aims to delay death. When I attended pharmacy school, the concept of healthspan barely existed, and they did not teach us how to assist our patients in preserving their physical and cognitive capacity. Today, the conventional space may acknowledge the importance of healthspan, but the standard definition – the period of life free of disease or disability – is insufficient. Holistic wellness pays far more attention to maintaining healthspan, or in other words, the quality of life.

Lifespan and healthspan are not independent variables, but rather tightly intertwined. The actions taken to improve healthspan will almost always result in a longer lifespan. For example, by increasing muscle strength and improving cardiorespiratory fitness, there is a reduction in the risk of dying from all causes by far greater magnitude than could be achieved by taking any combination of medications. The same goes for better cognitive health. Another related issue is that longevity, particularly healthspan, does not fit into the business model of the current healthcare, or "sick care," system. There are few insurance reimbursement codes for preventive interventions.

More broadly, longevity demands a paradigm-shifting approach to medicine that directs efforts toward a proactive approach to improving healthspan – and doing it now, rather than waiting until a chronic disease has taken hold or until cognitive and physical function has already declined. This needed change is not coming from the medical establishment; it will happen only if and when patients and healthcare providers demand it.

For most of my retail pharmacy career, I was a Pharmacy Manager, meaning I wore two hats, with sometimes opposite perspectives and obligations. As I transitioned into home care and focused on business operations, this led to another observation stemming from the nature of financial risk analysis. Minor, seemingly insignificant risk factors can compound and lead to an unstoppable situation. Chronic diseases work similarly, building over years and decades. A new way of thinking about chronic diseases, their treatment, and how to maintain long-term health, is to avoid their onset, or to divert from the path of affliction. Our strategies must change to fit the nature of these chronic diseases, with their long, slow progression.

All these combined experiences piqued my curiosity. As a fundamental aspect of human nature, curiosity motivates us to seek new knowledge, is the foundation of personal growth, and triggered my research journey into longevity and holistic wellness.

Being exposed to another way of thinking and changing my beliefs could only happen if I was willing to alter my convictions. Being set in my ways, this was not something easy for me to do. This trait works well in the regimented environment of retail pharmacy, but not so much when it calls for being open-minded. However, having conviction does not imply that anyone should avoid changing their mind when circumstances change. When confronted with new information, it becomes necessary to step back, question established practices, and reevaluate previous beliefs.

Paradigms shape our perception and understanding of the world. They serve as mental maps that help us interpret the information we encounter, influencing our personal and professional viewpoints. Developing a new evidence-based, foundational health paradigm presents a significant challenge, especially when it requires questioning conventional approaches and long-held doctrines. But by doing so, we can cultivate a paradigm that serves as a north star, guiding us toward optimal health, wellness, and longevity.

Utilizing my foundational knowledge in science and the core principles of human biology, I delved into the complexity, interdependence, and coordinated nature of the biochemical systems that sustain life. Things go wrong when we deviate from living in harmony with nature or in balance with ourselves and our environment. Disease and accelerated aging are not mistakes. They are our body's best attempt to deal with dire circumstances. Health and longevity are our natural states, but only if we understand how our bodies are designed to work best. We have extraordinary nutrient-sensing pathways essential to understanding how to eat to avoid disease, activate robust health, and live for a long time.

Consider an unhealthy plant. What is the best way to aid its recovery? Rather than administering medicine to the plant, the focus should be on addressing its environment. Ensuring the plant receives the appropriate amount of sunlight, water, and nutrient-rich soil becomes essential in restoring and maintaining its health. It is crucial to comprehend these factors' interactions and interconnected nature to understand the potential consequences when our human biological systems experience imbalances. Understanding how to create or restore balance, living with greater energy and youthfulness, and extending lifespan and healthspan is possible.

Rather than focusing solely on symptom management through pharmaceutical intervention, I now recognize the limitations of such an approach. I began to see how the conventional medical system strives to achieve a drug-induced state of homeostasis by manipulating test scores within predefined "healthy" ranges. However, it becomes evident that merely adjusting these results with medication does not address the underlying factors contributing to illness. Relying on drugs to regulate functions obstructs the body's natural ability to self-regulate and adapt to stressors, leading to a superficial improvement in biomarkers rather than genuine health. On the other hand, by pursuing lifestyle transformations, we can achieve a range of benefits beyond improvements in test scores. This comprehensive approach positively affects physiological markers, enhances the overall quality of life, and empowers individuals to take charge of their well-being.

Along with the shift in my paradigm, I also had to embrace a new mindset, an updated perspective, and a cognitive approach. Our philosophy continuously influences us, shaping our thoughts and actions, and is rooted in beliefs concerning our health, abilities, and potential. A fixed mindset believes fundamental qualities are unchangeable and views learning as threatening. On the other hand, a growth mindset thinks these qualities can be developed and improved over time and sees learning as exciting.

My evolving mindset regarding the now-recognized importance of sleep is a perfect example. For years, I overlooked this aspect of my well-being to my detriment. Embracing the mantra "I will sleep when I am dead," I took pride in staying up late during pharmacy school and my retail pharmacist career. I thought sleep was for lazy people, and nobody's end-of-life regret was to have slept more. Now, I understand that prioritizing sleep is necessary for optimum health, and I understand the significance of quality sleep on our physiological repair processes, especially in the brain.

Looking back at those two dark and stormy nights were specific moments that would shape the trajectory of my life, marking the commencement of a profound journey of self-discovery and transformation. As I embarked on my research and exploration into the realm of holistic wellness, I observed a striking pattern among numerous practitioners. Many shared a common background and narrative, compelled to find solutions for themselves or their loved ones when conventional medicine fell short. Like them, my unique story has shaped my personal and professional path, leading me to where I am today. However, unlike the others, I cannot point to a single moment for my transformation. Instead, my journey is an evolution. It is like being a passenger on board a massive ocean ship with momentum built up in the years of conventional medical practice and living an unhealthy lifestyle. Therefore, it took significant time to slow down to a stop and make a course correction.

In my many years as a Pharmacy Manager, I worked hard and enjoyed a prosperous and comfortable life. I was successful in my career, financially secure, surrounded by a loving family, residing in a beautiful home, able to travel and enjoy vacations, and partaking in various activities and interests. I was a high achiever who thrived in a high-stress environment in college and as a pharmacist. I was so focused on success and giving up so much of myself to care for others that I did so while sacrificing my health.

When looking back, I now realize that it started while attending college, when making poor dietary choices and forgoing workouts became ingrained habits that formed an unhealthy lifestyle over time. It worsened after graduation, as I became a full-time pharmacist in the high-workload, high-stress corporate environment of "do more with less" that was managed by numbers and metrics. I constantly multitasked and faced deadlines throughout my work days. I worked a standard 42-hour workweek, and stayed late to complete the necessary work despite an hour-long commute one-way. I also had all the household responsibilities on my time off from work. It had become customary for me to skip meals during extended shifts, with my only breaks used to drink a Pepsi. I was coping by choosing mostly unhealthy, processed food and eating excessively while escaping into a favorite book, magazine, or TV show.

Despite being a healthcare provider with extensive knowledge of disease risk, self-care was at the bottom of my priorities. I ignored my slowly rising weight gain and the red flag warning I received when hospitalized with a hypertensive episode. After discharge, I took high blood pressure medication, a solution that matched my mindset at that time. During that period, I felt the invincibility of youth, and believed that time was boundless. I continuously made plans to make changes, but always postponed them to a future date, a vague "someday, soon" when the timing was better, or an event had passed. I focused on building a successful career to provide for and care for my family. Prioritizing others seemed like a compassionate choice. However, the truth was that this mindset impacted my loved ones, whether I acknowledged it or not.

A common saying is that a journey of a thousand miles begins with the first step. But if we take the first step in the wrong direction, we will end up further away from the desired destination. The first step in my journey to better health was exploring the information that resulted in a shift in my paradigm and mindset, to ensure that my first step started in the right direction. The second step, and the one most people fail to complete, is making the necessary course-correction to change the trajectory of my life. I did so by applying the knowledge and taking action, one single step at a time.

The most significant change I needed to make was to no longer be a mere passenger on the ship, being carried along passively on a dark and stormy night at sea. I was now well-informed, medically literate, clear about my goals, cognizant of the true nature of risk, and ready to make important decisions. I was willing to alter ingrained habits, accept new challenges, and venture outside my comfort zone. I decided to actively participate and confront my problems, rather than ignore them until it was too late. In my new story, I was no longer a passenger on the ship; I became the captain. The time was now to set a new course.

To prevent being overwhelmed by the amount of information or having paralysis by analysis, I needed to detach myself and zoom out to gain a broader perspective. Taking a bird's-eye view of my situation provided a unique vantage point, the ability to see the landscape around me and the bigger picture beyond just my health challenge. By looking at my life from multiple angles, I achieved clarity. Specifically, I discovered my success when I examined my life through the lenses of health (holistic wellness), wealth (business principles), and time (attention management). I incorporated ancient wisdom, particularly Stoic philosophy (values and virtues), and modern advancements (science and technology). Most importantly, as I zoomed back in with this new perspective, I began to hold myself accountable and with a new purpose. As ship captain, I am responsible for my overall well-being.

Oftentimes we get caught up in what is optimal. And since we are all so busy and need more time to do what's optimal, we do nothing. Instead of an all-or-nothing approach, I began by embracing the powerful concept of making continuous improvements, which is the practice of making incremental daily changes with the belief that they will lead to significant progress over time. It emphasizes gradually adjusting everyday habits and behaviors rather than pursuing meaningful, distant goals. While these minor improvements may not seem impressive or noteworthy in the short term, they accumulate and compound over time, resulting in substantial advancements. By consistently making choices that are just one percent better each day, the cumulative effect can lead to being 37 times better after one year. Numerous studies support the idea that the most significant improvement in health and reduction in mortality risk occurs just by starting, taking an initial step. Excellence does not require a monumental effort nor incredible doses of willpower and motivation, just the discipline for small, manageable tasks, as mastery follows consistency.

I began with a small, simple, sustainable yet difficult change, customized to my situation. After years of indulging daily in my primary weakness, my challenge was eliminating Pepsi and Pringles, my kryptonite. Instead of looking at the desired health outcome, I focused on the process, making it through just one day at first, then on to consecutive days. Once my streak started, I then concentrated on not breaking the chain. The days extended into a week, weeks turned into months, months into years, and the unhealthy food habit has remained firmly in the past.

Through similar consistent efforts, perseverance, and discipline in diet, exercise, and meditation, as I write this, I am proud to say that I am in the best shape of my life and feel fantastic. The net result is that I weigh less now than in college, having lost approximately 75 pounds and eight inches in pants size. My blood pressure is under control. I do not take any medications. I do not say all this to brag, but as encouragement that anyone can transform their health using this strategic plan and tactics that I persistently used, enabling me to change my life's course by taking advantage of the power of momentum in this new and improved direction.

Looking ahead to my later years, I have shifted my goals beyond retaining just the minimal abilities measured by ADLs. I want more out of life than simply the absence of sickness or disability. I desire to thrive in every way throughout the latter half of my life. As I age, to accomplish these ambitious goals and maintain an active lifestyle, I must diligently uphold the fitness foundation already achieved.

After achieving this personal transformation, and because I figured it out, my passion is helping others do the same. I knew I had to find a way to share what I have learned in my evolution with as many people as possible, especially those in helping professions and caregiving roles. Sifting through the overwhelming volume and conflicting advice is among the most difficult aspects of this exploration. The more I learn, the more I discover that my research journey remains ongoing.

At the time of publication, I am in the preliminary stages of developing the framework toward fulfilling my mission as a navigator in charting a course in unknown waters and empowering others in their implementation. My intention is not to tell anyone exactly what to do, but to contribute to their education, knowledge, and self-enlightenment. While there is abundant information, the challenge lies in formulating a clear, actionable plan and the discipline to follow it diligently and consistently.

The most important message I can communicate is that we must take an active role to improve and preserve our health. Anyone willing to proactively take control, and sit in the captain's seat, will have the power to fulfill their life purpose, pursue their passions, and become the best version of themselves.

"The best time to plant a tree is 20 years ago. The second best time is now."
– **Ancient Chinese Proverb**

We often find ourselves deferring change, pushing it off to a point in the distant future. We subconsciously convince ourselves that transformation will occur after reaching a particular milestone or the start of a new period. For years, I was trapped in a cycle of procrastination, entangled in a web of excuses and justification that kept me bound to my familiar and comfortable routine. I constantly lived a few steps ahead, believing I would make a change, take control, and prioritize my well-being, but not until the next day. However, this mindset is detrimental, keeping us fixated on the past and constantly focused on the future.

It is important to remember that the past is unalterable, and the future is uncertain. Yet, within this truth lies the potential for transformation, where our destinies take shape. Recognizing this, I broke free from the allure of tomorrow, by embracing the power of the present moment to shape my future. Embrace this timeless wisdom, break free from the chains of procrastination, and seize the limitless opportunities that lie before and within all of us.

Take action, now.

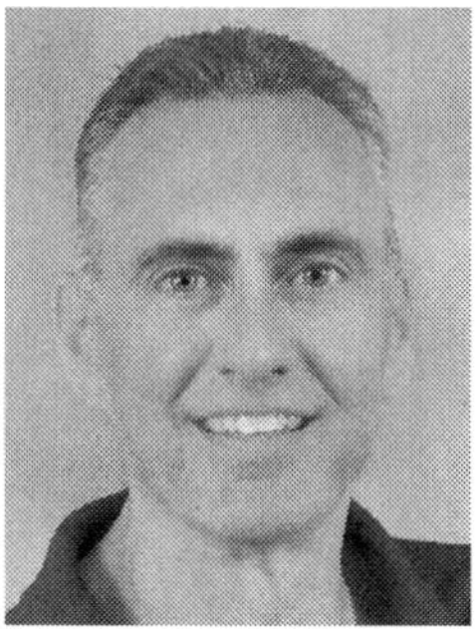

ABOUT ROGER BENEDETTI,

RPH, BPHARM

Roger Benedetti is a healthcare professional, wellness strategist, educator, writer, and speaker. He is the founder and President of Hibernian Home Care, an award-winning accredited agency providing various medical, rehabilitative, and supportive services.

Before becoming an entrepreneur, as a multi-state board licensed Pharmacist, he spent 25 years at a major national retail pharmacy in various roles in direct patient care and management. Over the years, he received numerous recognitions, including Pharmacy of the Year and Most Valuable Peer, and a commendation from the New Jersey Board of Pharmacy. In addition, Roger was a preceptor for pharmacy students and obtained various certifications in Diabetes, Immunizations, and Medication Therapy Management.

Roger developed an awareness working in these professional settings that the battle with chronic diseases wages on, despite modern medical interventions. He witnessed the failure to address the underlying causes. Roger's vision is a paradigm-shifting approach that transforms what is presently considered alternative or holistic into the mainstream, making it the conventional approach to healthcare and wellness.

Roger underwent comprehensive training at the STORRIE Institute™, where he learned how to integrate holistic wellness principles and modalities, such as healthy lifestyle recommendations and functional medicine, into his practice as a clinician. Roger is on a mission to help busy professionals, especially those in caregiving roles, who struggle to balance their careers, family, and health by implementing personalized strategies to create ownership with discipline and empower them to navigate their own course toward achieving their goals and optimum wellness.

Inspired by his personal health transformational journey, Roger found his passion for assisting others in achieving similar results. Drawing upon his enthusiasm for research and problem-solving, Roger aims to guide individuals to navigate the overwhelming volume of conflicting information, fulfill their life purpose, pursue their passions, and become the best version of themselves.

Roger is a professional college basketball Public Address Announcer at Monmouth University and has worked games at numerous large arenas.

www.RogerBenedetti.com | Roger@RogerBenedetti.com |
LI: @roger-benedetti

RESTORED

By: Suzette (Sue) M. Bornemann,
RN, MSN, APNP, FNP- BC, CSWWC

"He restores my soul; He guides me in the paths of righteousness for the sake of His name."

– Psalm 23:3

Stripped of everything I thought I was supposed to be, I realized that I would give up everything I own to have my health. A rare neurological disorder called idiopathic intracranial hypertension made me unrecognizable. I developed severe activity intolerance, vision disturbances, chronic pain in my head and neck, daily dizziness, and delays in processing speed. This progressed to periods of left-sided weakness, facial paralysis, slurred speed, and periods of loss of consciousness. Anxiety and depression invaded my world, and my mental health declined. But God. God gave me so much during this time. An understanding of who is for me, who sees me for me, and nothing else. During this time, I came to recognize the person in the mirror.

Idiopathic intracranial hypertension (IIH) is a rare neurological disorder. It occurs when too much cerebrospinal fluid (CSF) builds up in the skull, causing pressure on the brain and on the nerves in the back of the eyes (optic nerves). The most common complications of IIH include vision loss, vision changes, headaches, tinnitus (ringing in the ears), neck pain, and shoulder pain. The cause of this disease is unknown, yet many specialists suggest weight loss as the key intervention to managing this debilitating condition as obesity is highly correlated with IIH.

Oddly enough, I had lost 20 pounds in the months prior to developing symptoms of IIH. I was perplexed as to why I developed this condition, given the expert recommendations for weight loss to reduce symptoms. I read every research article I could find to help me understand why this might be happening to me. I purchased and read one of only two books dedicated to teaching people with this disease. I learned that venous congestion (or abnormal cerebral outflow caused by narrowing of the veins in the brain) is also strongly correlated to IIH. Months into my journey, I had a brain scan that specifically looked at the veins in my brain. My veins were found to be severely narrowed. I was relieved to find out that an anatomical issue was discovered and that I might be a candidate for a procedure to open the veins. Unfortunately, I had to fight for this procedure while taking medications for this disease that did not help and actually caused severe side effects. I had to fight because the doctor I was seeing did not believe that surgery would help me because the welling in my eyes wasn't bad enough. I was extremely frustrated.

As the weeks passed into months, my symptoms worsened. I developed severe activity intolerance. Activities like washing the dishes caused a sensation of increased head pressure, which exacerbated the blurred vision, dizziness, and painful paresthesias (numbness and tingling). I became so sensitive to light that I needed to cover all the windows in my house and put a cloth over my eyes when my husband took me to medical appointments. I couldn't look at a computer screen or my phone for fear of the searing pain that would develop in my eyes and head.

Unfortunately, the swelling in my eyes didn't change, and I still could not get a referral to simply talk to a surgeon about my concerns. I started to distrust the people who were supposed to help me.

I was in severe pain and was excessively fatigued. I could not think straight or speak normally. I was unable to exercise. I couldn't work. Even though I believed that further weight loss was not going to help with my IIH symptoms, I hoped it would. Besides, I was still considered morbidly obese with a BMI of 36 and comorbid hypertension and high cholesterol. I needed to strive for a healthy weight, but the dilemma with IIH had been figuring out how to lose weight when I was essentially bedridden.

I began to despise my body more than ever. I could not rely on my body to cooperate with me in anything, let alone weight loss. For as long as I could remember, my body image was that of self-hate. I hid myself from my husband, not allowing him to brush his teeth while I was in the shower. The lights always had to be off during sex, and I needed to be under a blanket. He told me I was beautiful, and he loved my body. As the tears flow right now, I recall my disbelief and the nasty things I said to myself internally.

Throughout my life I had been told I was fat or not thin enough when I was at a normal weight. I have always had to work hard at maintaining a healthy weight. The only time it was easy to lose weight was when I was ill or recovering from surgery. When I was diagnosed with hypothyroidism, I lost 40 pounds by simply treating the disease with levothyroxine. I remember the comments from family and friends: "Are you losing weight? You look great." What I heard was "It's about time – you have always looked like a fat, lazy, slob." I hated my body. I hated that others felt they had the right to comment on my body. Then the ease of weight loss from treating hypothyroidism wore off, and the pounds piled back on. I was disgusted by the exponential expansion of my body, and I didn't love myself enough to do anything about it.

IIH caused my body to betray me. As a survivor of physical and sexual assault, my struggle with self-hate became more difficult when the paresthesias started to affect my vaginal area and my breasts. One morning, I was messaging the neurologist about this. As I was typing, I noticed that I was becoming weak. I took my blood pressure – normal. I hit "Send" and got up to use the bathroom. I struggled to walk a mere 20 feet. My legs felt like they were made of lead, my vision was a haze, and there was excruciating pressure in my head. When I came out of the bathroom, I stopped in the kitchen and just couldn't move any further. My husband guided me to a chair, where I lost consciousness for 20 minutes. This became the first of many similar episodes. I hated my body even more. The medication I was prescribed for IIH was poison to me. I was contending with a decrease in kidney function, increased acid levels in my body (metabolic acidosis), and hypokalemia (low blood potassium). My memory worsened, and my thought processes continued to slow. Nothing in this world helped and I was not getting the surgical referral I thought I needed, so I prayed fervently in desperation.

> *Father God, please heal me from this awful disease. I pray that You will be done, but I want to be healed! You created us to be without infirmity. You created me in Your image, and You are so powerful and mighty. I am just a fat woman with a dysfunctional body, and I cannot do this without YOU. Please! Please heal me. In Jesus' name I pray for you to hear my plea.*

So, He did. He healed me by His will. He healed me of the self-hatred of my body. I began to hear His whispers of love.

Daughter, you are beautifully and wonderfully made in My image. You are created of Me in LOVE. I know you by name. I know every hair on your head, and I know how you hurt. You will be healed, and you will glorify Me.

God healed my heart and the way I see myself. I still battle the symptoms of IIH, but despite the activity intolerance, I did not gain weight and did lose some. I was healed of self-hatred and issues with body image. I managed through the pain of migraine. I continued to praise God because He taught me how to love myself unconditionally. I needed to be reminded of that love more than ever, because if I can't love myself as much as God loves me, how will I get through this difficult time? How can I ever follow my calling?

Throughout my career, I have felt called to support others dealing with issues I can personally identify with. I saw myself as an overcomer. After all, I am a nurse practitioner. I was a single mom at the age of 17, and I put myself through college. I did not let the pervasive nature of familial alcoholism, substance abuse, and mental health issues stand in my way. I conquered chronic fatigue syndrome and myofascial pain related to fibromyalgia. I survived. I did it. I am strong and I did not need any help until December 2018. That's when I fell into a deep depression, and my life was in danger. I cannot explain the details, but will say that I learned that I could not protect others from the things that happened to me and that cut me to the core. Desperate for help, my husband brought me to a church, where an amazing man of God shared the Gospel in a way I had never heard. On Tuesday, December 4, 2018, I surrendered my life to Jesus.

In my new life, God slowly revealed Himself to me. I learned more about Him, and realized that my life goals had revolved around creating a respectable resume. I saw myself for what the world saw. I saw myself as an independent, goal-oriented nurse practitioner. I needed to learn more, do more, and make more. I went through most of my life not knowing my true identity as a dependent child of God.

So, what does all this have to do with my journey in becoming a Certified STORRIE Wholistic Wellness Coach™? In 2022, my dear friend Jenny shared with me her family's journey with Functional Medicine. Her five-year-old daughter Elena had completed hair tissue mineral analysis (HTMA) testing, and her Functional Medicine provider recommended supplements to detox her from the high levels of heavy metals. Jenny shared that her personal exposure to heavy metals through a vaccine may have contributed to Elena's heavy metal toxicity. As a Western medicine-trained provider, I was skeptical. I observed as Elena progressed in her treatment; the symptoms of concern resolved. Elena was weaned off the supplements. Success!

At the end of that summer, the family incurred a serious traumatic event that sent everyone in the household reeling. The stress had a significant negative effect on Elena. Her tonsils enlarged, and she periodically stopped breathing while she slept. She developed symptoms consistent with autism spectrum disorder and absence seizures. Then Jenny felt a hard, swollen lymph node on one side of Elena's neck.

Elena was taken to her primary care provider. Labs were normal. An ultrasound of the lymph node and the EEG were both reassuring. The neurologist suggested that Elena was experiencing migraines. The otolaryngologist (ear, nose, throat specialist) recommended a tonsillectomy. While Elena was being evaluated by the Western medical providers, she had resumed treatment for heavy metal detox. Her Functional Medicine provider reassured Jenny that the tonsils and lymph nodes would reduce in size and that the symptoms consistent with absence seizures and autism would resolve when the detox was complete. Additionally, Elena was also expected to be relieved of headaches. Her parents decided to forgo the tonsillectomy, and I remained skeptical of the detox protocol. But you know what? The detox worked. Sweet little Elena is thriving!

The results are astounding, and I want to help others achieve optimal wellness through the most natural means possible. Plus, I want something I can never have in a busy primary care practice ... the ability to love people the way God intended. One thing I haven't shared yet in Elena's story is the faith that it took to stay on course. As the traumatic events unfolded and the concerns for Elena's health grew, God was sought first. It was His wisdom that guided my friend and her husband down the path of Wholistic Wellness™ that ultimately saw Elena healed. It was also God's wisdom that healed the pain of the trauma the family experienced that summer. No surgery, no synthetic medication, no therapy. It was faith, prayer, natural foods, and targeted high quality supplements that made the difference. That is something that Western medicine cannot do.

It was my faith in God that prompted me to seek certification as a Wholistic Wellness Coach™. When I decided to participate in the STORRIE Masterclass, I asked God for a very specific sign to confirm that this is the direction He was leading me to. He answered with an emphatic YES, and the incubation period of Trinity Wholistic Health, LLC began.

Trinity Wholistic Health, LLC will focus on helping individuals overcome symptoms of depression, anxiety, and post-traumatic stress disorder by supporting brain health. My vision is to be known as a caring, trusted, and respected source of wholistic wellness services such as hormone balancing, heavy metal detoxification, and nutritional support. It is my mission to inspire hope and contribute to the health and well-being of others by supporting individual aspirations through wholistic healthcare practices and the transformative love of God. God restored me to the hopeful person I was intended to be, and now I love the image in the mirror. With that love comes an understanding that optimal wellness is not the absence of disease, pain, or infirmity. Optimal wellness is the purest form of love for oneself that allows personal grace and mercy. Optimal wellness is the confident assurance in any circumstance that with Christ's love, we have no need to fear the present or the future.

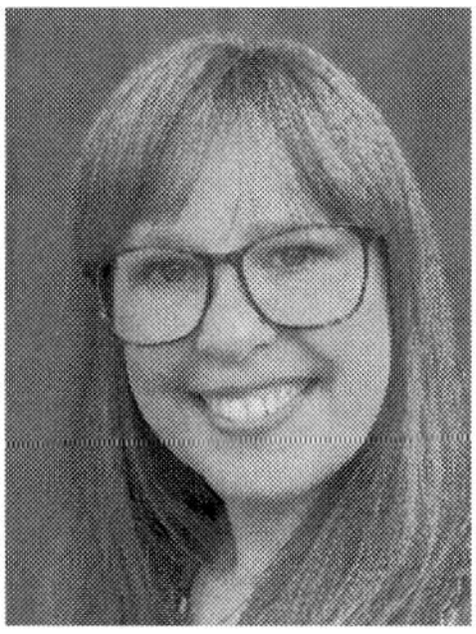

ABOUT SUZETTE (SUE) M. BORNEMANN,

RN, MSN, APNP, FNP- BC, CSWWC

Sue is a Christ-Centered Board-Certified Family Nurse Practitioner. She is currently enrolled in STORRIE Institute™ to become Certified STORRIE Wholistic Wellness Coach™ (CSWWC).

Sue has overcome numerous negative effects of trauma through prayer, nutrition, and hormone balancing. Upon her own transformation, she founded Trinity Wholistic Health, LLC, and intends to focus on helping individuals overcome symptoms of depression, anxiety, and post-traumatic stress disorder by supporting brain health.

Prior to developing her wholistic wellness practice, Sue worked within the traditional western medicine model. Her interests focused on mental health, trauma, and women's health. She supported numerous men and women in their recovery from traumatic experiences and in achieving a healthy love for self. She led multiple committees focused on healthy relationships and was a revered expert sexual health panelist for numerous programs. Sue has been published in the Eagle Herald and has authored curriculum and educational materials in the areas of human growth and development, relationships, and sexual health.

Volunteer work includes initiating a faith-based trauma recovery program with her husband, serving as a sexual assault advocate, supporting individuals with substance use disorder, coaching baseball for children and adults with disabilities, and serving in multiple ministry roles. Sue and her husband were foster parents.

People who know Sue describe her as kind, nurturing, and charitable. She and her husband, Jon, have an endearing relationship rooted and grounded in Love as defined in 1 Corinthians 13: 4-7. Sue believes the foundation of living well lies in understanding who we are as children of God. If you ask her what she does for a living, she will tell you "I praise God".

TrinityWholisticHealth@gmail.com | FB: @Trinity Wholistic Health

OUR BODIES SPEAK TO US, FIRST AS A WHISPER

By: Dr. Janine Brathwaite,
PHARMD, CSWWC

"If you listen to your body when it whispers, you will never have to listen to it scream."

– Unknown

The whispers I once ignored were now deafening screams demanding to be heard.

My first visit was to the dermatologist in 2018, when I suffered severe breakouts on my face. This was the first alarming sign in what became a series of warnings that my body would give over the next five years. I also was seen by the gynecologist and had tests performed to rule out polycystic ovarian syndrome (PCOS) and other hormone-related diseases. I would continue treatment with the dermatologist for two years with little improvement.

In January of 2020, I was involved in a car accident, which caused severe back pain for months. Following six months of physical therapy, the pain resolved. By the summer of 2021, the pain returned due to prolonged periods of sitting at work. During the pandemic, I was seen by a rheumatologist and orthopedist to assess the chronic pain and swelling in my hip and knees and the numbness and tingling in my arms. Standard diagnostic tests were performed, and the results were all normal. Despite X-rays, MRIs, and mounting medical bills, I still had no answers. I tried to ignore my symptoms, and began to rationalize them as the side effects of being a former Division I track athlete who sustained multiple injuries over the years. Ignoring these symptoms, or as I came to affectionately call them, "whispers," would be the catalyst in the perfect health storm that lay ahead.

In the spring of 2023, I found myself in the emergency room, after being referred by urgent care, due to an abnormal cardiac rhythm with inverted T waves. Despite visits to four different medical specialists, my symptoms continued to worsen, and my frustration at the lack of answers was at an all-time high. In addition to the bodily symptoms, I also suffered with severe brain fog, anxiety, and depression. I became apathetic as I now struggled with work and life in general. I wondered if I would ever get to the root of my problems. I knew something had to change if I had any chance at restoring my health.

The traditional and disjointed practice of evaluating my symptoms per respective health specialty had failed to produce any tangible results. Western medicine often looks to diagnostic tests to rule out or confirm the presence of disease, but this practice alone falls short in truly assessing the whole condition of the patient. The current healthcare model reinforces this practice by often requiring confirmatory tests before treatment is rendered or even covered by health insurance. We treat the test results not the patient! Symptoms are often rationalized and othered when the test results fail to confirm a diagnosis. Despite a positive antinuclear antibody (ANA) test and visible joint swelling, both the rheumatologist and I remained unclear about the root cause of my continued joint symptoms. My erythrocyte sedimentation rate, C-Reactive Protein (CRP), and complete blood count (CBC) were normal.

A different approach to addressing my symptoms and health in general was needed. I began researching holistic wellness, and hoped that the answers would be found in a more comprehensive approach in assessing my symptoms and entire body system. I learned about alternative diagnostic tests and treatment modalities, such as hair tissue mineral analysis (HTMA), mineral rebalancing, heavy metal analysis, and cellular detoxification. I also explored non-pharmacologic treatment options such as meditation and cognitive behavioral therapy for stress management and nutritional support. I also met with a hormone specialist to gain a better understanding of hormone dysregulation and the adverse effects on the body. For the first time in almost five years, I was hopeful about finally getting some answers.

My own health crisis and path to healing were my initial reasons to pursue Wholistic Wellness and to become a Holistic Wellness Practitioner. I met countless women who shared their health struggles and frustration with the traditional healthcare approach; I knew we were not alone. As I delved deeper, I found an entire community of women suffering in silence, trying to cope with similar and unexplained symptoms. I knew that healing myself with the aid of holistic wellness would not only provide the long-sought answers for myself but would be instrumental in changing the way we assess and treat our patients. Now, my "why" was much bigger than me.

For as long as I can remember, I wanted to be a doctor. As a child, I loved *Doogie Howser, M.D.* in my teenage years and *ER* and *Grey's Anatomy* in adulthood. These shows provided the narrative of what it meant to be a doctor; someone devoted to caring for and healing others. I held that altruistic view well into my late teenage years, but watching my cousin and her husband suffer through medical school provided a jolted reality of what being a doctor truly entailed. I decided then that a less hectic and more balanced life would be my goal. Growing up in Barbados, island living was a mix of hard work yet a vibrant appreciation for rest, beach days, and quality of life. Our holistic approach to life and health was ingrained in me. A teaspoon of honey and lemon was the go-to for a sore throat; Angostura® bitters, fresh ginger tea, and a minuscule dose of brandy cured any stomach ache; fresh coconut water rehydrated me on an exceptionally hot day; alcohol-soaked cotton balls under my armpits and in my socks broke many a fever before Tylenol®; and the Barbadian gold standard treatment for chest congestion and colds was covering your head with a towel while inhaling a boiled concoction of onion, garlic, turmeric, cinnamon, bay leaves, and menthol crystals. Sea moss and ginseng were a staple part of the diet, and a freshly picked soursop from the neighbor's tree provided vitamin C and antioxidants in the purest form. Back then, our diets were simple and still unsullied by the influx of American fast-food chains that would arrive after 2010. The food was real and fresh, and it nurtured the body the way it was intended. Muscle soreness and injuries were treated by warm saltwater baths, massages, strength, and mobility exercises, and stem therapy when needed. Medications were generally a last resort. Many of these holistic treatments, though not validated by Western medicine, have been bolstered by their undeniable results, many of which I can personally attest to.

At 18, I attended the University of Wyoming on a track and field scholarship. I graduated on May 9, 2009, with my Doctor of Pharmacy degree, and was filled with so much hope and enthusiasm for the career ahead. I first interned at a major retail chain in 2007 and would go on to work as a retail pharmacist for four and a half years.

During my time in retail, my perception of healthcare in America completely changed. I was on the front line of healthcare but had little time to truly care for my patients or hold even simple conversations with them. My days were filled with time-assessed metrics, weekly prescription budgets, daily vaccination totals, and countless profit-targeted programs disguised as patient care. The few meaningful patient encounters I had confirmed for me that holistic patient care was not only needed but deeply desired by my patients.

One such encounter was with a gentleman in his early fifties who wanted to get off his blood pressure medications. At the consultation area, he inquired about alternatives to medications. I advised him to speak with his doctor before making any changes to his medications, but I spoke with him about the importance of proper nutrition and exercise as parts of a healthy lifestyle. Almost four weeks later, I called him about his prescription but instead was informed by his wife that he was hospitalized with a stroke after his blood pressure spiked to 240/150. I wondered if an intervention sooner would have made any difference in his health outcome.

Another patient encounter involved a 29-year-old man who was recently diagnosed with type 2 diabetes. He came to the pharmacy with his prescription for a meter and testing supplies. I remembered him from visits to the pharmacy a few years back when he picked up his father's medications. He always had a pleasant disposition, and was one of the few customers who would ask how my day was going. At the consultation window, he expressed his fear of dying young from diabetes like his father. He said that nearly everyone in his family had diabetes and that he didn't want this disease to dictate his quality of life or fate. This was one of the most heart-breaking conversations I had with a patient. We were the same age, but our health conditions were in stark contrast. I was in great physical shape and had no health conditions. I spoke to him about the important roles of proper nutrition and exercise in maintaining a healthy lifestyle. He politely asked me if he could ask a personal question. With his acknowledgment of my professional boundaries, I apprehensively responded to his question. He asked my age, but prefaced the question by indicating that I didn't need to disclose the actual number but merely indicate if I was over 30. He remarked about my youthful appearance and physical fitness. I spoke to him about my personal fitness routine and encouraged him to join the gym. Over the next six months, I watched him transform as he lost 40 pounds and resolved his diabetes. Monthly visits to the pharmacy became friendly health check-ins, with him reporting on his progress with weight loss and changing his diet. He credited me with his success, but I quickly assured him that he deserved the credit for taking control of his life. This was by far the most meaningful patient encounter I ever had, and it was further confirmation of what holistic patient care embodied.

As the years passed, I became more conflicted about the career path I had chosen. I witnessed glaring inadequacies in our approach to patient care while the health of my patients declined. I felt powerless to change the narrative as the daily demands of running the pharmacy were ever-increasing. On the eve of my 30th birthday, I made the decision to resign from my full-time pharmacist position. I transitioned from retail to the Medicare specialty department for one of the largest health insurance providers in the country. I welcomed this change and was enthusiastic about the opportunity to engage in more clinical care. Although the job was more aligned with the vision I had for myself as a practitioner, it failed to provide any opportunities for comprehensive patient care in several areas. The first six years on the job were professionally challenging but allowed for a better work-life balance.

It was now March 2020, and I witnessed the world thrown into chaos because of the global COVID-19 pandemic. Life and work had taken on a new sense of urgency, and the ever-increasing work demands began to blur the once-clearly delineated work-life balance line. As a work-from-home pharmacist, I found myself frequently working outside of my designated work hours just to meet the increased work demand. My morning routine transitioned from meditation and exercise prior to work to me logging on as early as 6 a.m. to get a head start on case reviews. Case reviews had increased from 25 per day to 35 per day. I began to feel the strain and disconnection within myself. Most days, my team and I worked well into the night, just to keep pace with the demand as case reviews now exceeded 35 per day. Six months into the pandemic, my body began to exhibit signs and symptoms of distress. My sacred morning routine was almost nonexistent, my nutrition had declined as my weekly food preparation had fallen by the wayside, and I developed insomnia from working late into the night, haphazardly meeting my colleagues online at 1 and 2 in the morning to complete urgent case reviews.

Life had become a hurried mess and I was drowning, but like most healthcare providers, we all felt a sense of obligation to our patients. As 2021 was ending, my body was in full-blown crisis mode. I had mostly ignored the signs and symptoms that had existed for almost a year. My back pain returned, I gained 25 pounds from stress eating and lack of exercise, and I precariously tethered on the brink of a mental breakdown. Having ignored all the warnings, I was in a state of burnout. I was physically, mentally, and emotionally exhausted. On May 27, 2019, the World Health Organization (WHO) defined burnout as the following:

> "… An occupational phenomenon 'conceptualized as resulting from chronic workplace stress that has not been successfully managed.' Burnout is typically characterized by three dimensions.

According to the WHO, doctors can issue a diagnosis of burnout if a patient exhibits three symptoms: feeling depleted of energy or exhausted; feeling mentally distanced from or cynical about one's job; and problems getting one's job done successfully. The WHO notes that burnout is to be used specifically 'in the occupational context.'"

I was exhibiting all three symptoms of burnout. According to the *New England Journal of Medicine*,

"Burnout manifests in individuals, but it's fundamentally rooted in systems. And health worker burnout was a crisis long before COVID-19 arrived. Causes include inadequate support, escalating workloads and administrative burdens, chronic underinvestment in public health infrastructure, and moral injury from being unable to provide the care patients need. Burnout is not only about long hours. It's about the fundamental disconnect between health workers and the mission to serve that motivates them."

I requested a 10-week leave of absence to address my own health and to tend to my sick mother. My travel plans for Christmas of 2020 were upended by the pandemic. A visit home was both a necessary reconnection and a medical intervention, as my mother's cancer prognosis worsened. I returned to the United States a few weeks later, with a heavy heart, clearer mind, and lighter body frame. I lost 20 of the 25 pounds I had gained the previous year. I resumed a regular exercise routine, improved my nutrition, and worked with my therapist to establish a healthier mental and emotional state. Upon returning to work, I was thrust back into the chaos. I struggled to maintain the balance I had established for myself while I was away. That year was the most difficult for me personally and professionally because I had a relentless urge for a profound change in my professional career. I continued to grapple with my professional discontent, and again, the symptoms I had temporarily quieted were again rearing their heads.

March of 2023 was the breaking point. I ended up in urgent care one morning after feeling exhausted with a lingering discomfort down my back. After a full examination, the doctor informed me that I needed to go to the hospital by ambulance. After I was discharged, I wore a continuous cardiac monitor for a month. At the conclusion of the cardiac monitoring, my cardiologist assured me that my heart was fine and that my condition was likely brought on by stress. On the one hand, I was relieved by his findings, but on the other hand, I was further frustrated by the continued decline in my health. During the months preceding my hospital visit, I worked late nights trying to meet my daily productivity requirements of 38 cases per day and the mandatory additional cases requested. The workload seemed never-ending, and I continued to struggle at work, physically and emotionally. My discontent with work heightened after my request for short-term disability was denied. I was frustrated by the process and further disgusted by the assessment of the severity of my depression and anxiety, given the supporting documentation provided by my therapist of 10 years. My personal responsibilities of caring for my cancer-stricken mother were stressful enough, but the added job-related stress made the situation untenable. I was hardly sleeping or eating, and I was exhausted. Western medicine relies on evidence-based medicine to diagnose and treat health conditions, but it does little to fully address the root cause of disease. I liken this approach to tending to the leaves and branches of a tree with rotting roots.

According to Albert Einstein, the definition of insanity is "doing the same thing over and over and expecting different results." My attempts to manage my health-related symptoms had been unsuccessful time and again. Western medicine and traditional diagnostic tools failed to provide any definitive answers regarding my bodily symptoms, and the mental health assessments and documentation requirements from my employer for short-term disability exacerbated my stress. Mental health services provided by my therapist were the essential thread that held me together throughout my health crisis. I exhausted all traditional treatment modalities except psychoactive and pain medications, because I knew that my symptoms were manifestations of a deeper issue that could include cellular neurotoxicity (due to exposure to chemical, environmental, and dietary toxins that result in a cascading effect in all body systems), chronic inflammation, hormonal dysregulation, and autoimmune disease, to name a few. My decision to become a Functional Wellness practitioner was born out of my own desperation to get to the root cause(s) of my health conditions and to restore my health. Following COVID, the growing need for holistic wellness was simply undeniable as the incidence of chronic health conditions skyrocketed.

According to the National Association of Chronic Disease Directors' Commentary on Chronic Disease Prevention in 2022, "Many routinely miss or ignore their body's warnings about the onset of a serious chronic disease or are unable to receive preventive care due to social or economic barriers. The result is poor collective health quality in the country that spends much more on healthcare than anywhere else."

According to the Centers for Chronic Disease Prevention and Health Promotion (NCCDPHP), "Six in 10 adults in the U.S. have a chronic disease and four in 10 have two or more."

For all the reasons listed above, I decided to start my own Wholistic Wellness practice called The LIFE Co., which stands for The Living in Full Equilibrium Company. Wholistic Wellness has always felt like home to me. In a world where symptoms are often ignored or not validated by Western medicine, it becomes more important that we fully embrace a holistic approach to healthcare. The check engine light that illuminates in our car serves as a parallel to symptoms exhibited by our body when something is not right and requires attention.

My mission at The LIFE Co. is to empower individuals on their path to holistic wellness by addressing the root causes of their symptoms before chronic disease develops. I believe that true wellness requires that we live in a state of balance in the mind, body, and spirit. Through a proactive and integrative approach, we strive to uncover the underlying imbalances and triggers that contribute to the manifestation of warning symptoms. By addressing these root causes, the goal is to prevent progression to chronic disease and to enable individuals to live their fullest and healthiest lives.

"Your body can heal itself of anything if you provide it the right environment to do so."

– Unknown

References

1. Chronic Diseases in America. https://www.cdc.gov/chronicdisease/resources/infographic/chronic-diseases.htm. Published December 13, 2022. Accessed July 7, 2023.

2. Commentary on Chronic Disease Prevention. National Association of Chronic Disease Directors. FS_ChronicDiseaseCommentary2022FINAL.pdf. Accessed July 7, 2023.

3. Zhang, Y. Cell toxicity mechanism and biomarker. *Clin Trans Med* 7, 34 (2018). https://doi.org/10.1186/s40169-018-0212-7

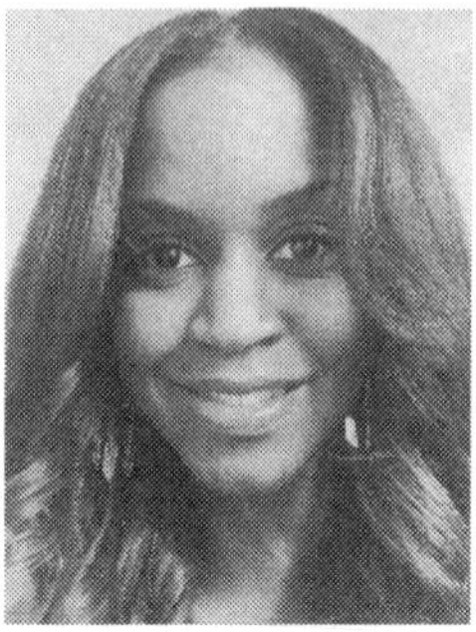

ABOUT DR. JANINE BRATHWAITE,

PHARMD, CSWWC

Dr. Janine Brathwaite is the creator of LIFE Co. Wellness and is currently pursuing certifications in Functional Medicine, Personal Training and Nutrition, and a Certified STORRIE Wholistic Wellness Coach™ (CSWWC) from STORRIE Institute™.

Dr. Janine immigrated from Barbados to attend university on a Division I Track and Field scholarship. She graduated with a Doctor of Pharmacy degree in 2009. After graduation, she served as Pharmacy manager for a major retail chain for four and a half years. She transitioned to a major health Insurance provider and served as a Clinical Pharmacist and Board-Certified Geriatric Practitioner for over nine years.

Her departure from corporate life was prompted by her own health challenges, that were exacerbated by work-related stressors during the COVD-19 pandemic. Unresolved by traditional medical practices, she sought answers in Wholistic Medicine. Her unresolved health conditions and denial of Family Medical Leave and short-term disability were the driving forces in creating LIFE Co. Wellness.

LIFE Co Wellness is a holistic wellness practice focused on helping women, aged 30 to 50, restore their health and vitality through cellular detoxification. The program will utilize lab testing to identify root causes of chronic inflammation, impaired metabolism, vitamin and mineral deficiencies, heavy metal toxicities, hormonal imbalances and premature aging.

Dr. Janine is passionate about helping women restore their health and reclaim their lives. She sees herself reflected in women everywhere as she too struggled to resolve her own health challenges. She will continue to champion the voice of women and fiercely advocate for holistic health care solutions to support their complex body systems. She is a firm believer of the body's innate ability to heal itself if we create the right environment.

Pharmfitinnovations.com | Info@lifecowellness.com |
IG: @Fitbodypharmd

THERE HAS TO BE A BETTER WAY THAN THIS ...

By: Dr. Alicia Bryant,
PHARMD, CFMS

"Behold, I will bring to it health and healing, and I will heal them and reveal to them an abundance of peace and truth."

– Jeremiah 33:6

Throughout school as a child, I grew up drawn to math and science. Being able to see an equation solved and find evidence that something was fact was very satisfying. It just made it all make sense. When it came time for my senior year of high school to start, the decision for a career path became center focus. How can I take my strengths and use them to serve others? Initially, I wanted to go into psychiatry as a way to help others on their life journey. To my surprise, my dad said "Nope, pick something else!" due to the length of time needed to complete a terminal degree and the instability of the post-graduation job market in his estimation. While researching alternative careers in the healthcare field, pharmacy was mentioned and I went with it. After all, I could still get the opportunity to coach people on their health ... just in a different way than I initially imagined. Sure ... let's do this!

Off to New Jersey I went with my wild ambition and grand intentions for the future. Six years at Rutgers University did not disappoint. I learned so much about the potential to educate, empower, and unleash the potential within others … even if that meant using medications as the primary tool to assist. Ok, this could really be great.

Soon after my graduation and indoctrination in the "real world," I quickly realized that these ideas would remain just dreams due to the constructs of modern-day medicine. I witnessed doctors spending less and less time with patients, creating a huge gap in education and the understanding of their health. I literally found myself spending more time with the patient in the counseling window, in the clinic office, or on the phone with them than they ever get with their provider … and of course I'm more easily accessible. Gone are the days where patients were educated in the office and later that information confirmed by the pharmacist. People have less and less faith in or are simply unable to access their provider and are turning to Google and social media as their guide. Doctors don't have the time to spend challenging the fads or inaccurate information, or even dig deeper to find the root cause of why we are so sick in this wealthy nation. Forced by low reimbursement rates to see as many patients as possible during the course of an office day, the visits have gotten shorter, the questions asked and answered minimized, confidence in healing evaporating, and frustration levels mounting. Health insurance costs more and appears to deliver less. We have become a sicker people, even though America is one of the wealthiest countries in the world. We have begun to lean on quick fixes, and have abandoned the traditional design of asking questions, appropriate testing, and putting in the work to determine what is causing the patient to be out of balance.

Here enters the concept of holistic wellness, which helps to liberate people from the confines of Western medicine. Rather than focus on taking another medicine to "cure what ails you," it takes a hard look at the total person, seeking to answer the question, "*Why* are you ill?" You have physical, emotional, spiritual, and mental pieces that go into your overall being. Dealing with only one part of the puzzle will not help get to the root for true healing. For example, several years ago, I went to the doctor due to experiencing reflux symptoms every morning. Not once did the doctor ask about my food or beverage intake, my exercise regimen, or anything else. I was quickly prescribed a popular medication used to treat reflux. For a few weeks, I took the medication and started to feel a little better but not overwhelmingly so. However, I started doing my own investigation, noting my intake via a food diary. *Orange juice*, which at the time I was drinking every morning, was actually what was bothering my system. Once I stopped drinking it, there was no need for the medicine any longer. What the heck?!?!?! It was a much simpler and cheaper answer to my problem that could have been addressed sooner with a little more investigation from the provider.

Recently, I had a customer ask for an over-the-counter product to help her husband deal with a side effect of his new medicine and health diagnosis. After asking a few pointed questions, it was found the patient was already on a prescription medication in the same drug category that the wife was requesting! It's so easy to get into duplication of therapy when you are winging it and relying on commercials, search engines, and your neighbor for solutions. We also spent time discussing ways her husband could improve his health by moving around and simple diet changes. The wife was grateful for the information and relieved to know there were other alternatives.

I counseled a woman for 10 minutes about her caffeine intake during the day. Not surprisingly, she was having subsequent trouble sleeping each night. She really had not thought about it. The experience was eye-opening, and gave her renewed hope for her energy levels if she put limits on her intake and monitored her timing. Providing a few small, measurable, and attainable changes can truly empower and reroute the trajectory of one's life. Inviting you to be an active participant in your health, and determining which goals are most important for you to crush, is a very different approach from what we are used to. This is what holistic wellness stands by, and it has become the tool I can use to help others.

Feeling like you are on the merry-go-round of appointments, prescriptions, medicine, energy drinks, and muffin tops with no progress? Think you are unworthy of having and feeling better? You don't have to stay stuck. This is the reason why I founded Find And Ignite Transformational Hope (FAITH), a holistic wellness company designed to help you get to the root cause of your specific issue. I would love to work with you and create a plan to help you reach your wellness goals with lifestyle modifications, movement, and necessary supplementation. There has to be a better way than this … and there is!

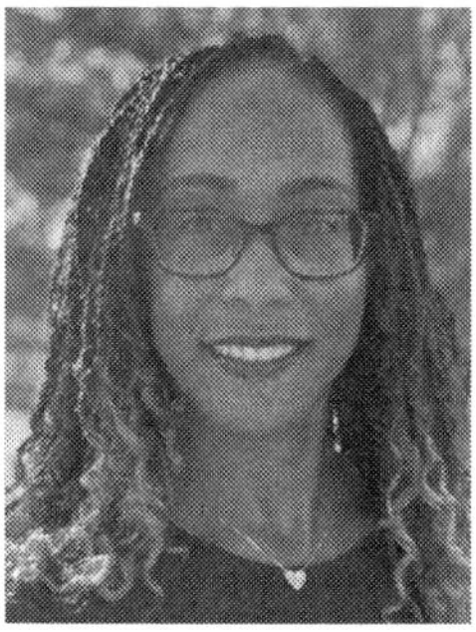

ABOUT DR. ALICIA BRYANT,

PHARMD, CFMS

Dr. Alicia Bryant is a licensed Pharmacist, Certified Functional Medicine Specialist™ (CFMS) from STORRIE Institute™ and the founder of Find And Ignite Transformational Hope (FAITH). She graduated from Rutgers University and has been practicing pharmacy in various clinical roles and settings, to include Pharmacy Benefits Management, the Veterans Administration, academia and specialty clinics. She holds a Masters of Science degree in Human Nutrition from the University of Alabama. She is also a proud veteran of the US Air Force.

Within her holistic wellness practice, FAITH, Dr. Bryant utilizes functional medicine strategies to help adults who feel stuck in their personal health journey by identifying the root cause and establishing attainable goals. Her approach to improvement involves a combination of nutrition, exercise, supplementation and other appropriate lifestyle modifications.

Outside of her professional duties, Dr. Bryant enjoys working out, traveling, watching college football and helping out with student ministries at her local church.

www.dralicia.co | support@dralicia.co | FB: @Alicia Masters

JOURNEY TO PROFESSIONAL ALIGNMENT: FINDING HEALING AND SUCCESS THROUGH HOLISTIC HERBAL MEDICINE

By: Dr. Marina Buksov,
PHARMD

"First the word, then the plant, and lastly the knife."
– Asclepius of Thessaly

Life is a combination of destiny and personal actions, but the journey is equally important. Our perspectives and reactions shape our lives. I remember when I first embarked on my wellness journey, and how confusing it was to navigate the healthcare system, even as a licensed healthcare professional myself! Not having any guarantees of safety or efficacy, in a model that's built on showcasing exactly that in an evidence-based way, was absolutely shattering for my worldview and everything I'd worked so hard to accomplish in my pharmacy career up to that point.

On the precipice of graduating and starting my career, I became plagued with mysterious illnesses. I was going from specialist to specialist, and agreeing to more and more invasive therapies, including polypharmacy, procedures, and surgeries – which, in retrospect, did more harm than good. I felt like I was running out of options. I then decided to seek alternative modalities, and found that I was responding to some of the more gentle approaches. I spent thousands of dollars and hours on self-care, self-help, and various forms of healing, from herbs and acupuncture to energy work. (How ironic it is that insurance covered only surgeries and drugs but not holistic approaches, which were much cheaper in comparison.)

Even though I ultimately found there is no "magic bullet," I started to take more responsibility for my own health and to cultivate a relationship with and deep trust of my own body wisdom. This is why I do the work I do and advocate for holistic health and professional alignment.

My background is in the allopathic pharmacy field, and I hold a PharmD from St. John's University. I graduated *Summa Cum Laude* in 2013, distinguished by Rho Chi and Phi Lambda Sigma honor societies, and tied for third highest GPA for the entire College of Pharmacy and Health Sciences graduating class.

Bushy-tailed and wide-eyed, I was super-excited to put my newfound knowledge into practice. However, I soon discovered that I wasn't particularly aligned with any of the myriad of pharmaceutical paths available to me.

None of the diverse rotations or internships I'd experienced as a student really called to me. Neither did pursuing additional training in a residency or fellowship program. I should've been at the top of the world, proud of my achievements and ready to jump into the next chapter … but I found myself in a major conundrum and at the verge of depression instead.

A mere few months shy of graduation, I realized that I might have just made the biggest mistake of my life.

Allow me to backtrack a little bit and tell you about my life leading up to a turning point that changed my entire professional and personal trajectory. My own health issues guided me toward my calling in the health field. It all started with digestive problems during my childhood in Ukraine, marked by gas, bloating, and stomach pains. Moving to America introduced me to a new diet, which worsened my weak gut and led to a diagnosis of Irritable Bowel Syndrome (IBS) in high school.

College brought its own challenges. Burping became a persistent issue, leading to an endoscopy that diagnosed a gastric ulcer caused by *Helicobacter pylori*. Aggressive medical treatment, including antibiotics and proton pump inhibitors, did not provide relief. However, advice from my pharmacist led me to probiotics and herbal alternatives, which finally eased my symptoms. This experience sparked my interest in herbal studies.

As I approached graduation from pharmacy school, I began experiencing unexplained symptoms. Excessive tearing in my eyes affected my confidence. Determined to secure a successful future, I attended a conference, but felt overwhelmed and unprepared for the positions I interviewed for. The pressure to fulfill my parents' expectations weighed heavily on me. My discomfort was amplified by my teary-eyed appearance, affecting my performance. Eventually, I realized that my inner self did not align with my actions. After deep self-reflection, I turned down a job offer and accepted a position at a local pharmacy, although it still didn't feel completely right.

My skills called on me to be a drug expert, but I wanted nothing more than to see people thriving without drugs ... because what I learned in pharmacy school was so much more than drug therapy! I also learned about the value and power of nonpharmacological approaches as first-line therapy, no matter what the disease state.

And what I experienced working in the retail setting, and being a patient going through the healthcare system myself, reinforced this deep truth. The reality as I saw it was that the health system was rigged for failure and a wasteful use of resources.

We were focusing on changing clinical outcomes and endpoints utilizing targeted drug therapy very late in the game, rather than identifying earlier markers of health and disease. We were overly focused on prescribing a "pill for every ill," rather than focusing on prevention and public health.

We systematically followed the guidelines, but did not question how the guidelines were established in the first place, and by whom, and who they really served. We started on the healthcare path to help people with selfless compassion, but found ourselves powerless and lacking autonomy to make any real changes in the one industry that wasn't supposed to be corrupt.

While working at the retail pharmacy, I continued to search for answers regarding my health issues. I explored various alternative therapies, including acupuncture and naturopathy, and delved into the world of herbal medicine. Through my personal experiences and research, I discovered the power of a holistic approach to health, which considers the interconnectedness of the mind, body, and spirit.

During this time, I also encountered patients with chronic illnesses who were seeking relief beyond what conventional medicine could provide. I realized that my knowledge and expertise as a pharmacist could be utilized in a different way – to support individuals on their healing journeys. I began sharing information and resources with these patients, empowering them to make informed decisions about their health.

I identified with my patients and deeply cared about finding better, less invasive, and more sustainable solutions to support their health. I believed with all my heart that there was a better way, and wished I knew more about alternatives so I could educate others and make an impact.

So, the next logical step for me was to stop beating myself up for choosing the wrong major and getting a useless degree.

Instead, I understood that I learned powerful lessons, not in spite of becoming a pharmacist, but because of it. Being behind the counter and dispensing countless amounts of medications that did little to address root causes, and had lots of potential risks and toxicity associated with them, was what pushed me to seek deeper answers and solutions. So, instead of starting over in a completely different industry, I chose to repurpose the skills that I already had and channel them in another direction.

As my passion for natural health grew, I knew that I needed to make a change in my career. I boldly decided to leave the comfort of the retail pharmacy and pursue my true calling. I launched my platform "Raw-Fork" to educate and inspire others to take control of their health through natural means. Through my blog, social media channels, and workshops, I started spreading the message of holistic wellness.

Of course, this didn't happen overnight. I worked in the retail pharmacy setting by day, and spent thousands of dollars and hours gaining additional skills and planning an exit strategy from an unfulfilling and unaligned role by night. But this pursuit for a better way beyond the "straight and narrow" was not done alone. At first I attempted to figure it all out on my own, but eventually realized I needed support and guidance.

I'm grateful for it now, because it has made me a better coach and mentor but … I made a *lot* of mistakes along the way that I learned from later. Once I worked up the courage to ask for guidance, the path was still challenging, but no more challenging than school or anything else I pursued in life. I hired a number of mentors and coaches to help me bridge the gap in the areas I was not proficient in. I mean … when I started, I knew *nothing* about business.

After meandering through various training programs in health coaching, nutrition, and Functional Medicine, I was drawn to explore an alternative way of practicing pharmacy. It was something that never occurred to me, even though I was always fascinated by blending natural therapies with modern medicine. I just never thought to become an alter ego of traditional pharmacy by literally turning to the roots of our profession, which indeed are steeped in herbalism (excuse all the puns)!

So, I explored a local herb shop, and arranged for an unpaid internship. Fascinated with all the plants and their properties, I decided to dive even deeper, and pursued a formal three-year clinical herbalism program.

Finally … I felt at home here. Everything I'd learned in and outside of pharmacy school had come together in the herbalism field. Moreover, I found myself at a great advantage over my classmates in regards to digesting and absorbing the material. Knowing the jargon of pharmacy, and having the understanding of pharmacology, gave me a huge leg up.

It was like pharmacy gave me the strong backbone, and now I was layering in a variety of diverse colors, textures, and shades of herbal therapeutics. What I learned about plant medicine went way beyond reducing plants to their mechanical parts and extracting the coveted pharmacological activity from various constituents.

I was immersed in learning about the energetics, the qualitative properties, the botany, and the very intricacies of the spiral lattices that govern every living being in the natural world. I felt connected to all of the brilliant humans who studied and classified herbal medicine before me – because this knowledge was universal and transcendental.

In addition to learning how and what plants can do for us, I found myself gaining a deeper understanding of the interdependence of all living ecosystems and the importance of diversity in the natural world. Seeing that we are all connected and in constant relation to each other ultimately gave me a grasp of how to live a meaningful human existence.

While I was working and studying, I was also building my business in the background. I started tinkering with various offerings in my services, seeing clients 1:1, and building a website. I co-wrote and published an ebook, and grew my network of like-minded pharmacists. Eventually, I was interviewed by The HappyPharmD ... and that exposure opened the floodgates.

I wanted to pay it forward and show the next generation of pharmacists that it's possible to have a successful career as a natural-minded pharmacist, and began researching and interviewing others on this path. I created The Holistic Pharmacy podcast, featuring the stories and trajectories of pharmacists and other industry leaders of holistic, Integrative, and Functional medicine.

Before I knew it, more and more pharmacists inspired by my path started reaching out to me and asking to pick my brain ... and all of a sudden, people began asking to pay me for my guidance. At that point I saw an opportunity to continue paving a new path for many to follow after me.

As I continued building my business, my knowledge base, and relentless research, it became very clear that there was a demand for this work far greater than what I could supply alone. To fulfill the demand for holistic approaches to all the health ailments out there would require a movement.

All of this reminded me what fulfilling your purpose actually feels like, and I realized at that point there was no going back, only forward. I knew I would have a long road ahead of me, but the ability to compare how I felt working at the pharmacy – and the feeling I felt being able to serve my clients with autonomy – compelled me.

I had to figure out how to work full-time and take care of my family, while going through one program after the other, building all the tools and skills I possibly could around herbalism, as well as business. As if it wasn't hard enough to juggle all of that at once, we were in the midst of COVID-19, and I became pregnant with my second child.

And this chapter of my life introduced yet another health challenge. Two weeks postpartum, I started experiencing debilitating new-onset headaches. Little did I know, these headaches did NOT turn out to be migraines like I thought, but were symptoms alerting me to a very serious acute condition that could result in permanent neurological damage!

Instead of being in maternity bliss, I found myself hospitalized for a week with a surprisingly severe case of cerebral venous sinus thrombosis. I underwent extensive testing and imaging, was put on a cocktail of IV drips (including painkillers, which I reluctantly agreed to knowing all the risks of tolerance, and my personal history of two unmedicated births), and had emergency endoscopic sinus surgery.

Though I received excellent care from the brightest minds in New York City, for which I'm eternally grateful and to which I owe my life (thank you NYU Langone Health!), my stay was far from restful. I was desperately trying to keep my breast milk supply up via pumping, even while exhausted from all the procedures and discomfort of being in an acute care setting. It was challenging to keep morale up, and to get any semblance of sleep.

The road to recovery had some bumps as well, with inflammation and pretty gnarly sinus healing processes (I'll spare you the details). But I literally had the will and instinct to survive in each given moment. With my husband not leaving my side, I made it through each passing challenge, one at a time. I took things slow, and got through each day with gratitude for getting to live to see another day.

It took a close call with death for me to realize the extent of how beautiful life is. It's all in the eye of the beholder. I wanted to keep going for the sake of my children, and my mission and purpose that is not yet complete here on Earth. So now I get to continue, with a renewed sense of balance and wisdom of yet another powerful lesson my soul is learning from my body's experience. I'm remembering that pain is inevitable, but suffering is optional.

Looking back on my journey, I realize that my health challenges were not just obstacles, but valuable lessons that guided me towards my true path. They taught me the importance of listening to my body, exploring alternative approaches, and trusting my intuition. They also highlighted the need for a more holistic and personalized approach to healthcare, one that considers the unique needs of each individual. They also instilled in me the wisdom to discern which tool to use when – and that we can and *should* integrate holistic and Western medicine. They each have a role to play in not only keeping us alive, but helping us thrive.

Finding my calling has brought me a deep sense of fulfillment and purpose. It has allowed me to combine my passion for natural health with my expertise as a pharmacist, creating a unique and meaningful career. I have witnessed the transformative power of following one's true path, and I encourage others to explore their own passions and listen to the whispers of their hearts.

To date, I have created a mix of high- and lower-ticket services, in the format of self-paced, real-time, virtual and in-person classes, workshops, 1:1, and group programs. I also craft herbal tea and tincture formulations, partner with other brands, and currently earn residual income from my virtual dispensary. And I even managed to run my first retreat in the middle of the pandemic – international to boot!

The path to get to where I am today was not easy, nor did I do it alone. For me to build my business on the side, launch it, and scale it successfully while juggling everything else required me to learn how to build my business around my lifestyle and other responsibilities that were non-negotiable. I invested over $100,000 in the last couple years on courses, coaches, consultants, and mentors in order to find ways to serve others with the knowledge, experience, and passion I had in the most efficient way possible.

That is how and *why* I pivoted to helping other pharmacists build their holistic practices while giving them the freedom and flexibility to work remotely part-time and, for some, full-time.

Through my education, coaching, and business endeavors, I help other pharmacists navigate the realm of possibilities of their own earning potential and pursuits. I have developed a systematic approach to train and support budding holistic practitioners. And because I have followed the path myself, I understand what it takes not only to step onto this path, but how to tread it much more efficiently.

And the reality is ... many have been conditioned to believe it's nearly impossible to pivot from the path they are on to a more holistic path that puts people over profits – let alone "successfully." However, the definition of success lies in the eyes of the beholder. My version of success has been a fluid definition that has been constantly morphing and evolving as I take aligned action steps that bring me closer to my next goal.

My journey is far from over. I continue to learn and grow, exploring new modalities, expanding my knowledge, and connecting with like-minded individuals in the field of natural health. I am grateful for the experiences that have shaped me and the opportunities that lie ahead. My hope is to inspire others to embrace their own journeys, trust their instincts, and find their true callings in life.

I encourage everyone to listen to their bodies, follow their passions, and trust the wisdom that comes from adversity. The journey to finding your calling may not always be easy, but it is a rewarding and transformative path worth pursuing. If any of this resonates, I'd love to connect and see if I can support you in adding in holistic practices to find your version of success.

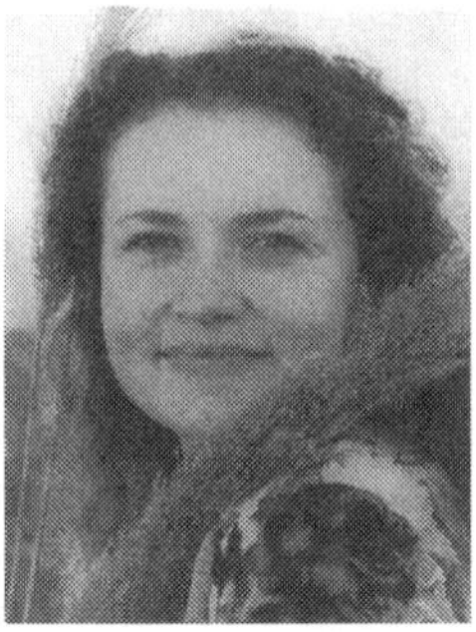

ABOUT DR. MARINA BUKSOV, PHARMD

Dr. Marina Buksov, PharmD, is a Functional Pharmacist, Clinical Herbalist, Mental Fitness & Health Coach, Herbal Educator, and lifelong learner of the Healing Arts. She is the creator of Build Your Holistic Herbal Practice course mentoring other healthcare professionals in clinical herbal as well as business skills. She leads the Herbalism Channel at RPhAlly to increase the utilization of herbal education for pharmacists.

Dr. Marina guides practitioners to rediscover their passion for medicine by expanding their mind and clinical skills to include natural, holistic, alternative and herbal medicine from which conventional medical practice originated! She believes in honoring plants as food and medicine for sustainable & sovereign health.

She is also a functional medicine pharmacist as part of PharmToTable telehealth platform, and the host of the Holistic Pharmacy Podcast. Dr. Marina uses her multidisciplinary background to educate patients about the least invasive and most natural methods for healing the spirit-body-mind. Her truly holistic approach helps women embody the best versions of themselves and lovingly celebrate the skin they're in.

When she is not studying, Dr. Marina likes to dance, paint, and tinker with various concoctions (tea blends, meals, DIY projects). She lives with her husband, two adorable kiddos and two mischievous kitties in NYC.

www.marinabuksov.com | marina@rawfork.com | IG: @marinabuksov

Subscribe to The Holistic Pharmacy Podcast

DOUBLE TROUBLE

By: Dr. Janelle Caruano,
BCIDP, PHARMD, CSWWC

"Ask, and it will be given to you; seek, and you will find; knock, and the door will be opened to you: for everyone who asks receives; the one who seeks finds; and to the one who knocks, the door will be opened."

– MATTHEW 7:7-8 NIV

Growing up in a house on a wooded lot can be awesome for a child, especially in autumn when all of the leaves are changing to vibrant colors of red and orange and falling from the trees. Raking leaves isn't a chore when the end result is an opportunity for play with the nicely organized piles. Many people can say they've shared laughs and memories of throwing leaves and jumping in the piles as children. Unfortunately, I can't say I share this same joyful memory, because during my childhood, I suffered from asthma and many environmental allergies. As a result, I missed out on the simple and little things in life like jumping in the piles of leaves, because I would develop severe congestion and coughing from such an activity. Any time someone who lived nearby would start burning leaves, my mom would call me in the house from playing outside, because even the smell of burning leaves would cause my congestion to worsen.

As you can imagine, coming down with a cold and getting sick was no fun either, let alone for a child struggling with asthma. My allergist prescribed for me breathing treatments, otherwise known as nebulizer treatments, at the age of 3, when I was first diagnosed with asthma and multiple environmental allergies. Thank goodness for the breathing treatments, because they were much needed, especially when I would spend countless times awake in the middle of the night with uncontrollable coughing due to my asthma. Despite this inconvenience during the night, I have fond memories of my mom trying to help pass the time by playing a game of *Trouble* with me, which almost always lasted about the amount of time it would take to do a complete breathing treatment with the nebulizer.

Even as a teenager, I used to struggle with the simple task of running in gym class, especially when it was time to complete the annual one-mile fitness test. I would dread this task, because I was usually one of the last ones to finish. My lack of lung capacity and endurance was an issue, as I was still reliant on the medicine that allowed me to breathe easier.

Yes, conventional medicine with the breathing treatments and inhalers helped me gain temporary relief for my asthma and allergies, but my parents also instilled in me the importance of holistic medicine. My mom often sought out alternative treatments and guidance for my asthma and allergies from the local health food store. I even started seeing a chiropractor at a very young age. As a result of my parents seeking healing for my condition, the holistic or Functional Medicine side has always been ingrained in me since I was a child.

As I grew older, my lifestyle changed, my eating habits improved, my level of exercise and overall wellness improved, and so did my asthma and allergies. My reliance on conventional medicine to help me breathe easier was fading as well. It was now only a rare occasion when I would need this medicine, rather than a common occurrence.

As a product of my environment and experiences, I knew pursuing a career in the health field was where I needed to be upon entering college. I started by getting my first real job in a retail pharmacy as a pharmacy technician at the age of 16. Working in the pharmacy was a great experience, because I was able to shadow and learn firsthand what being a pharmacist was like. I saw the close relationships the pharmacist formed with the patients and how well they knew the history of each person who was a regular customer at the store. Upon graduating high school, I had no doubt that pharmacy school was the path for me. For anyone squeamish at the site of blood, like myself, being a pharmacist was a great alternative to being a nurse or a doctor. Additionally, having grown up with close interactions with the healthcare system because of my conditions, healthcare was an attractive field for me to pursue. I decided to apply to pharmacy school, and was soon accepted as an undergraduate into the doctorate program with a guaranteed seat as long as I could maintain a certain GPA. While I was attending college, I began interning in a hospital pharmacy. I absolutely loved all of the knowledge base that could be applied in such a setting with critically ill patients to serve and help. This internship paved the way for my first job as a pharmacist in the hospital setting after graduating college. I truly felt like my six years of doctoral education was being put to good use as a Clinical Pharmacist in a hospital.

On my second day on the job as a brand-new pharmacist graduate, one of my bosses approached me and abruptly stated, "You need to pick a committee to get involved in." Since it was my second day on the job, I really had no clue what committees even existed for me to get involved in, so I asked what my options were. She proceeded to tell me one of the options was the Antimicrobial Stewardship Committee. That sounded like a good fit for me since I enjoyed infectious diseases while learning about it in college, and it also played a critical role in my childhood filled with respiratory illness. So I replied, "Sure, I will give the Antimicrobial Stewardship Committee a try." I have to admit that during that moment, I was actually taken aback by this forward statement from my boss, only to later realize I had her to thank. This person soon became a mentor for me while I served as the Antimicrobial Stewardship Pharmacist for the remainder of my hospital career. She pushed me to further my career in this realm of infectious diseases, and taught me the ropes about having a leadership position. I started precepting and teaching pharmacy practice residents about infectious diseases, and really took on a role as an educator for our department and the hospital in this specialty area. The momentum continued further, and I became a Board Certified Infectious Diseases Pharmacist. My motivation to help others even led me to create, implement, and run a new allergy-testing service at our hospital for those labeled with a penicillin allergy.

Regardless of these career accomplishments, I always felt that there was more I could be doing for patients. Yes, I implemented new services for patients in my specialty area and educated others, but I had to stick with conventional medicine because of the field I was in. Looking back, I realize now that something deeper inside me always wanted to help patients from more of a Functional Medicine perspective. I would think a lot about the immune system and even gut health, which was also closely integrated with my field of infectious diseases. It seems like "there's a pill for every ill" was the way medicine was prescribed, when I believe there is more that can be done to heal people with chronic diseases rather than bandage over the symptoms and create life-long dependency on medications. And so it was, after serving in the same hospital for 14 years after graduating college, I left the acute care hospital setting in 2022.

I am going to rewind a bit back to 2017, when the turning point and shift in my mindset really occurred. In 2017, I experienced "double trouble" and began managing allergy and asthma symptoms again, only this time it wasn't for me but for my 1-year-old son. He was diagnosed with respiratory syncytial virus (RSV) for the first time when he was just 6 months old.

Fortunately, given my experience with managing asthma and respiratory symptoms, I was able to keep him from being hospitalized because of it. This was only the beginning. He later suffered from RSV again, multiple bouts of croup that landed us in the emergency room, and constant congestion and asthma symptoms. It was a rare day when he wasn't a mouth breather from his nasal congestion. When he was a young toddler, he also developed eczema on both of his legs. He was seen by multiple doctors and allergists who gave him prescriptions for his asthma and allergy symptoms and steroid creams for his eczema. With my background as a pharmacist, I knew these medications were only going to treat the symptoms and not actually cure the underlying cause. I didn't want him to rely on asthma and allergy medicine for his congestion or steroid creams for relief from the itchy eczema for the rest of his life. I knew there had to be more. Yes, the steroid cream would help the itchy symptoms, but what was causing this to begin with? What was his body reacting to, and what was his skin trying to tell me with this eczema? The allergist decided to do a panel of allergy-testing skin pricks on his back. Needless to say, it was the most torturous experience, not only for a now-2-year-old boy but also for me, his mother. His whole back "lit up," and he reacted at least mildly to everything. I was instructed to avoid certain foods, start him on a bunch of maintenance medicine, and see how he did. How was I going to tell a 2-year-old who was already a picky eater that he couldn't eat some of the few foods he didn't have an aversion to? I wasn't happy with the answer the allergist had given and the maintenance medicine to help with symptoms. What about the healing cure? My son's immune system was broken, but what was specifically broken about it? I was determined to find a better answer, so I took him to see another allergist and explained his situation. Again, without any deeper answer, she also suggested the maintenance medication and creams for his itchy eczema, which I was determined not to use. I became even more frustrated after being dismissed by yet another doctor who wasn't taking the time to actually listen to what I had to say. It's one thing to "talk the talk" and say you are someone who listens, and it's another to actually "walk the walk." Here I was, longing for a doctor to walk the walk.

After feeling helpless and defeated, like when you know something is wrong but no one seems to have a better answer, I decided to take matters into my own hands and get to the root cause of my son's issues, who at this point was now 3 years old. This was the Functional Medicine side and holistic wellness approach ingrained in me kicking in. After doing my research, I began modifying my son's diet, and I added in some supplements and vitamins because I knew he was lacking in proper nutrients, especially with his picky eating habits. In a few weeks, his eczema started to improve. Occasionally, it would even disappear for a brief time, and I wasn't even using any steroid cream on it. I was persistent with my approach, and after a few months, his eczema was completely gone! His constant congestion was gone. My son was having days of breathing clearly out of his nose rather than his mouth, which wasn't the case even when I was giving him the allergy medicine. To this day, at the time I am writing this, I am glad to say he is a happy and healthy 7-year-old boy who is asthma- and allergy-free without the need for any chronic maintenance medication and no more steroid creams! It was the Functional Medicine approach of lifestyle modifications that helped to achieve this transformative outcome.

Fortunately, I have been asthma- and allergy-free as well for many years now, and I want to help others achieve this same improved quality of life through Functional Medicine. I know firsthand and understand the frustration of chronic congestion and allergies. I want to help others who have the same feelings that I experienced, who are searching for answers to their health questions and know there has to be more. I am here for those who want to dig deeper into their health and speak to someone who walks the walk.

The specifics of my story and my son's are unique to us, but the underlying message is the same and likely similar to many others' health stories. My story is a testimony that you have to listen to your gut. If you are a parent like myself, your gut instincts probably frequently kick in. The same should be said not only for parenting, but also for your health. Listen to your gut instincts. If you feel something is wrong or you know there has to be more, then dig deeper. If you feel there is something missing, then there probably is. Don't ignore your instincts and what your body is trying to tell you. Functional Medicine is that approach that seeks to uncover the root cause of illness and disease in order to provide the body the proper nutritional support it needs to heal naturally. "… Seek, and you will find; knock, and the door will be opened to you." Matthew 7:7 NIV.

Some may view the health experiences of myself and my son as a burden, but I don't, because everything in life happens for a reason and is often there to teach us something. My life experiences have been a blessing and building blocks of learning to pave the path for where I am today. I needed to have asthma and allergies as a child to become interested in the healthcare field and to help others with their health. My first job in a retail pharmacy when I was 16 gave me the career path to pursue pharmacy education. My college internship helped me realize I wanted to work in the hospital setting. My boss telling me to get involved in a committee my second day on the job pushed me to specialize in antimicrobial stewardship and infectious diseases. My childhood experiences with illness also gave me the interest to pursue this speciality. My drive to help patients suffering with allergies led me to create and implement an allergy-testing program at my hospital. My passion for infectious diseases motivated me to become board certified and to educate and share my knowledge with others when I began serving as a pharmacy resident preceptor. My experience as a pharmacy resident preceptor helped me develop the skills to effectively mentor and coach others. My son's health struggles provided for me the realization that oftentimes we have to be our own healthcare advocate in order to dig deeper and get to the root cause of someone's illness.

I am here today with these life experiences that have built upon each other and taken me from Board Certified Infectious Diseases Pharmacist to Certified STORRIE Wholistic Wellness Coach™ in the space of Functional Medicine. My experiences also inspired me to start my own business, HHW Lifestyle, LLC, where I can finally practice what I know about – and live by – health and wellness. The "HHW" stands for Health, Happiness and Wholeness, which are the focal points of my business. I am passionate about serving those suffering with chronic allergies so they too can experience the transformation to a better quality of life through personalized lifestyle changes like my son and I have. All of the experiences that I've been describing remind me of a 1903 quote from Thomas Edison: "The doctor of the future will give no medicine, but will interest his patient in the care of the human frame, in diet, and in the cause and prevention of disease." It was these lifestyle adjustments that produced the positive changes my son and I needed in our health for prevention of future asthma and allergy symptoms. These lifestyle adjustments were the missing links that we didn't get from conventional medicine.

If you feel like there is more to uncover, are ready to dig deeper concerning your chronic allergies, and are ready to take charge of your health and wellness, then please connect with me. At the center of HHW Lifestyle, LLC is care and compassion. I have an honest and vested interest in the well-being of my clients. I take the time to listen to my clients' complete health story, and use my knowledge and experience in the health and wellness field to formulate the best lifestyle plan for that individual. My vision for my clients is to experience a better quality of life. I want those I serve to feel their best so they don't have to miss out on living a fulfilled life anymore because of their allergies. I want my clients to find healing and inner peace, the **Health, Happiness, and Wholeness** they deserve!

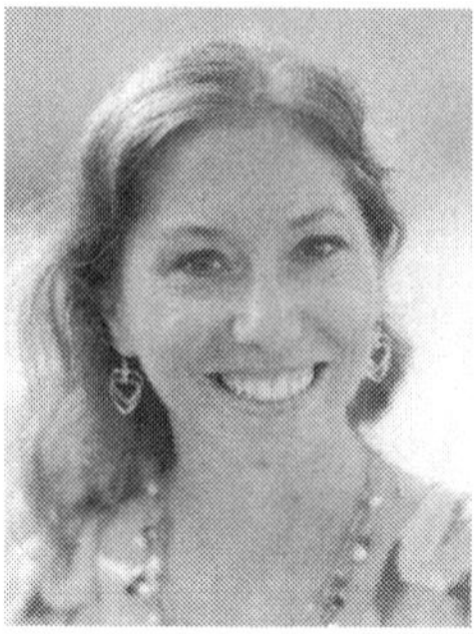

ABOUT DR. JANELLE CARUANO,

PHARMD, BCIDP, CSWWC

Dr. Janelle Caruano is a Functional Medicine Practitioner, Founder and CEO of HHW Lifestyle LLC, Certified STORRIE Wholistic Wellness Coach™ (CSWWC), Clinical Pharmacist Specialist with Board Certification in Infectious Diseases, Health Educator and proud mother of two. Dr. Caruano has spent the last 15 years in healthcare with a passion for allergies, the immune system and infectious diseases and understands how gut health has an impact on each of these areas, as well as overall body wellness. During her career, she has helped many patients with medication allergies through an allergy testing program she implemented and managed in the healthcare setting.

Dr. Caruano has served as a speaker and educator for other medical professionals on allergy testing programs, antimicrobial stewardship, and infectious diseases at conferences, symposiums and through newsletters. Her collaborative work and accomplishments have been published in the Delaware Journal of Public Health as well as being named the Pharmacist of the Year through the Delaware Society of Health-System Pharmacists in 2013.

With the gut being the cornerstone and gateway to overall health, Dr. Caruano helps middle-aged adults achieve improved quality of life by supporting optimal gut health as preventative medicine and encourages the body to heal through the utilization of nutrition and personalized lifestyle changes. Not only has she helped her patients, but she is a living testimony to transforming health through holistic wellness for both herself and her son's struggles with asthma and allergies. She has always had a drive and desire to help others and is excited to do so in a way she lives by and believes about health and wellness.

Dr. Caruano's vision is for her clients to experience the Health, Happiness and Wholeness (HHW) they deserve!

www.drjanellecaruano.com | info@drjanellecaruano.com |
FB: Janelle Caruano

FROM 3D TO 4D TO 5D: MY PATH TO HEALING BODY, MIND, HEART, AND SOUL

By: Dr. Lauren Castle,
PHARMD, MS

"The secret to having it all is knowing you already do."
– Author Unknown

Being that I am the founder and CEO of the Functional Medicine Pharmacists Alliance, it may come as a shock to hear that Functional Medicine isn't the "be-all and end-all" that I once believed it to be. When this modality transformed my husband's health in 2015, I was convinced that it was the solution to the healthcare crisis, so I started a master's degree program to learn all I could about this modality and bring it to the world. What I didn't know then is that over the next eight years, I would face many of my own physical and mental health challenges that would put this belief to the test, and it would only be further compounded by the most profound loss and grief I've ever experienced when my mom passed away at the age of 59. This journey brought me to the realization today that Functional Medicine was merely the gateway to a new path of higher and deeper levels of healing far beyond the conventional methods that I was initially conditioned to trust in as a pharmacist. If Functional Medicine was the gateway to this new path, psychedelics were the key that unlocked the door to a whole new world of Quantum Wholistic Healing™ for me.

3D Healing: My Background and Path to Pharmacy

As a child, I was quiet and curious, but brave and adventurous. I was also sick, *a lot.* I remember dosing out my liquid medications: pink antibiotics, orange antipyretics, and purple cough suppressants. I have a photo of me riding around in a red wagon with my oxygen mask on to receive nebulizer treatments. But despite my immune system challenges, I was an active, happy, and creative kid. I loved art, drawing, gymnastics, cheerleading, dancing, and singing just as much as I loved climbing trees, riding roller coasters, collecting bugs and crystal gemstones, and conducting science fair experiments.

Growing up, I went to a private Christian academy at our church until it closed its doors in 2003 and I had to start going to public school in eighth grade. When it came to my dream jobs, I wanted to be an artist, fashion designer, and model in third grade, a veterinarian in fifth grade, then a quantum physicist in seventh grade. In 11th grade, I got a part-time job as a technician at an independent pharmacy, and I knew I had found my vocational calling. Pharmacy was a great fit: I could help people without having to touch them, I'd get a doctorate degree in just six years, and it offered financial stability and job security, as pharmacist demand was at its peak back then.

It was also in 11th and 12th grade that I lived as my most authentic self: an "emo kid" with crazy "scene hair" who became friends with everyone and was a member of as many extracurricular activities as I could fit in my schedule: the school newspaper, robotics team, German club, photography club, choir, bible club, and church youth group activities like dance team, drama team, and praise team where I sang and played guitar. All the while I maintained straight A's in AP classes and capped off my senior year as Homecoming Princess.

But behind the diamond tiara and heavy black eyeshadow, there were struggles too. While everything looked perfect from the outside, my mom was suffering from alcoholism my entire life, and it affected our family deeply. Despite all my praying in church for her miraculous healing, it never came. As I wrestled with God, I internalized so much of the trauma that I didn't even know I was experiencing, and deep down I constantly felt like I wasn't a good person and that I was never enough. It was a feeling that would keep fueling my ambitious drive for perfection for the next 15 years.

Upon entering pharmacy school, everything changed for me. Classwork no longer came easily, and my new motto was "B's and C's get PharmD's." I stepped away from church and leaned into the party culture, but still maintained my drive for leadership roles and making friends in all the circles of campus. I was heavily involved in Greek life as a vice president for my fraternity Kappa Alpha Theta, served on Panhellenic Council, and was a recruitment counselor. In my third year, I became the first-ever ONU representative on the Student Leadership Council for the National Community Pharmacists Association. I was also nominated to the Pharmacy Council, Phi Lambda Sigma, Mortar Board, and Order of Omega.

At the beginning of my fourth year, I went to a fall fraternity party where I met and fell in love with my soulmate, and we've been inseparable ever since that night. We spent that first year visiting each other on the weekends. When we decided to move into an apartment together that summer, I needed to pursue a new internship, which is how I ended up at a large supermarket chain pharmacy. I chose this path thinking it would be helpful to gain new experience in a very different setting, and that I'd still go on to own an independent pharmacy. But after sharing about my positive experience in that first summer internship, and having my story published in the health and wellness email newsletter for the whole company, I realized that I had found a company I could grow with and impact millions of lives, potentially even the world. Upon graduating, I became a staff pharmacist and then was quickly promoted to pharmacy manager in Ohio, before my husband and I moved to Michigan for our jobs, and where our path to functional medicine would begin.

4D Healing: The Path to Functional Medicine

Many pharmacists and healthcare professionals end up on the Functional Medicine path in search of answers that conventional medicine hasn't been able to provide. That was our story in 2015, when a brochure showed up on our doorstep describing every symptom that my husband had been struggling with, including brain fog, fatigue, weight gain, anxiety, sinus issues, gut problems, and more. I thought we were doing all the right things to be healthy, like choosing whole wheat bread and skim milk according to the food pyramid as well as trying to sleep and exercise. I had exhausted every option I knew of as a pharmacist, outside of starting on prescription drugs that I felt would just cover up the symptoms. My husband decided to go to a weekend seminar to learn more before signing up for a 12-week all-inclusive program. After all the extensive labs and food sensitivity testing, the doctor uncovered my husband's root causes of candida overgrowth, gluten and dairy sensitivities, low vitamin D, and low testosterone levels. Within weeks of starting the professional grade supplements and an elimination diet, all his symptoms began to disappear, and he lost 20 pounds. He came out on the other side with a new lease on life. Being a supportive wife, I followed along with the elimination diet too, and quickly discovered the difference between feeling "fine" and understanding what optimal health truly felt like. But over the next eight years, my quest to pursue perfect health and evermore knowledge of Functional Medicine would simultaneously lead to my own burnout, and a new path of emotional and spiritual healing I never expected.

In 2016, I started an online program for my Master of Science in Human Nutrition and Functional Medicine at the University of Western States. While still completing my degree, I was promoted to clinical manager and then again to a market health and wellness director for my employer in 2017. In this new leadership role, my dream was to integrate a Functional Medicine approach in the retail pharmacy setting to transform the profession from the inside out. That dream nearly became a reality in 2019, when I got to meet members of my employer's executive leadership team and board of directors while leading a three-month home office project in conjunction with the new health centers being developed. My goal was to create a "healthy café" with nutritionists and medically tailored meals, all integrated with the multidisciplinary care team and the patient's shopping experience. But as quickly as the opportunity came, *poof* – it disappeared in an instant. Organizational leadership changes ended all projects and sent me back to my market director role in Ohio, but I came back with even more determination to change the profession, now from the outside in. In 2020, I started an LLC for the Functional Medicine Pharmacists Alliance (FMPhA) and created our membership website to begin the work of starting a movement to make Functional Medicine the standard of care through pharmacist-led clinical services.

Just a month after returning from my project and formally starting the FMPhA membership, my world turned upside down, not only because the pandemic hit, but also because my mom's health took a turn for the worse. Back in 2017, on the day I interviewed for the market director position, I found out my mom had been admitted to the ICU in the hospital and diagnosed with cirrhosis. I flew down to be with her for a month while I was between roles, and then brought her back up to Ohio a few months once she had stabilized. I spent the next four years as her primary caregiver through the revolving doors of hospitalizations and long-term care facilities, all while completing my master's, chasing my corporate dreams, and growing a national grassroots movement. The years 2020 and 2021 were by far the hardest; not only was I watching my mom's organ systems begin to fail, but unknowingly my own physical and mental health was deteriorating as well under all the stress. When my mom passed away on September 12, 2021, it was the final straw that led me to my own breaking point. No longer could I put the needs of the world before my own. It was time for a change in my life.

5D Healing: My Own Journey to Health and Wholeness

The first warning signs that something was off in my own physical health came much sooner than 2021. While pursuing my master's in nutrition, I had also become obsessed with dieting and exercising. I was working with a fitness trainer who had me tracking every macro on a 1,300-calorie diet and doing fasted spin classes three days a week plus lifting weights five days a week. I leaned out at 127 pounds and 16 percent body fat and put on eight pounds of muscle, but I also had been skipping my periods on birth control since the age of 17. This only added fuel to the hormonal fire. After a few nagging injuries from lifting and overtraining, I was finally forced to take a break from the gym when the COVID pandemic hit. When I went off birth control in September 2020, I expected my periods to return, but six months later, they still hadn't. A DUTCH test in February 2021 revealed low levels of estrogen and progesterone in the range of a perimenopausal woman. I began reading all the books I could on women's health, including *Period Repair Manual*, *Beyond the Pill*, and *Woman Code*. I cut out alcohol, started on a 2,500-calorie food plan to bring my body back into safety, and did acupuncture to stimulate the blood flow. It wasn't until a month after my mom had passed that my periods finally returned. It was like my body knew that we couldn't even think about ovulating until I was no longer a caregiver.

The second warning sign was in my mental health. Through 2020, no one knew what was going on, and we were all just trying to figure out how to survive the pandemic. But by the summer of 2021, we were mostly just adjusting to the "new normal." For me, though, nothing was normal. I had always been a high performer my whole life, and while I was making progress on my physical health and hormones, the Functional Medicine interventions weren't making much of a difference in my mental health. I had previously had a few instances of panic attacks in high school and college, but more and more, I was getting to the point where I couldn't walk into one of my pharmacies without experiencing a racing pulse and heart palpitations. I couldn't sleep because I'd be up all night rehearsing work conversations in my head. I'd sit at my laptop absolutely paralyzed by overwhelm as my inbox crept up over 200 emails each day. And as Mom's health got worse, I'd spend my early mornings visiting her and then crying in my company car as I commuted to my stores, worked up the nerve to go in, and put on a smile and pretend like I was okay.

My manager is ultimately the one who noticed that things weren't okay and suggested that I look into a mental health leave for myself, or at least family leave to take care of Mom. I had leveraged our 24/7 helpline a few times in moments of sheer overwhelm and sadness, and so I decided to set up a virtual appointment with a psychiatrist to get a professional opinion. It was a call that absolutely changed my life. After 32 years with a parent with alcoholism, I had never once been to therapy or talked to any professionals about what I was going through. The doctor suggested that I enroll in an intensive outpatient program (IOP). Before I even had the chance to make the decision to take a break from work, my mom passed away that Monday. I spent the next 10 weeks at IOP, three days a week for three hours a day of group therapy, sitting in the same seat that my mom sat in just one year prior. I learned a lot about mental health and myself as well as all sorts of coping skills through that process. I came out on the other side much better equipped to return to the working world and life as I knew it, but with a few key changes. I stepped down from my role as a market director and took on a new position working from home in social media marketing. It was a fun change of pace in an area I was passionate about and wanted to develop my skills in. I had plenty of clinical and operational experience, and now I could add marketing to my resume too. I worked in that role for 11 months, but by August of 2022, I felt the old familiar feelings of anxiety and depression creeping back in as work became more stressful, FMPhA was continuing to grow, and I was traveling extensively for both roles. I was still in therapy for maintenance, my physical health was fully restored, and all my labs were great. So why was I struggling with my mental health again?

As the approaching anniversary of my mom's passing grew closer, it was illuminating the hole in my heart that hadn't yet healed. Through a series of serendipitous conversations with three of my friends who all recommended psychedelics as a helpful tool in their own healing journeys, on September 11, 2022 I had my first psychedelic experience, and at long last was able to release much of the trauma I had been holding on to. This awakening of my own consciousness set in motion a new chapter in my life, one in which I could finally see the beauty in all the pain of the circle of life and death.

In February of 2023, I had an opportunity to spend 18 days in Costa Rica at Con Smania Retreat Transformational Center for back-to-back retreats, and I left with more than I could have ever imagined. By learning ways to achieve elevated states of consciousness, through breathwork, meditation, plant medicine, and shamanic journeying, I learned how to connect with my mom in spirit. Through this process, it all became clear the purpose of my struggles and hers as well. A few months earlier, when I was first making plans to come to Con Smania, I had an opportunity to invest as a member of the Collective, but at the time it wasn't financially feasible. Now, I had inherited my mom's estate, and a seat on the Collective had opened again for me to become a member. It wasn't even my own money – it was truly hers and her spirit that would make this dream into a reality. Through her legacy, I would be able to help others find peace, love, and healing so they too could be happy, joyous, and free.

One important thread through my story is that opportunities will come to you when you are ready for them. My journey to healing needed to happen in phases; to move from conventional to functional to energetic and spiritual. With each leap, plant medicines (both herbal supplements and psychedelics) and lifestyle medicines absolutely were the bridge to help create the mind-body-spirit connection needed to evolve. I find it so fascinating that faith and spirituality ultimately were the keys to higher levels of consciousness, which helped me discover my purpose through the story of my life. Perhaps others reading my story will be able to discover their own healing journey through the 15 years of growth I went through. For me, I've simply learned that prioritizing my own self-care and becoming the best version of myself ultimately helps everyone else around me too.

Conclusion

If you're a pharmacist or healthcare practitioner, I invite you to join us in the Functional Medicine Pharmacists Alliance (fmpha.org) to help grow the Functional Medicine movement that will transform healthcare from the inside out. But I also invite you to join me personally at Con Smania Costa Rica (consmaniacr.com) to do your own inner work that will be required of you to create the true conscious awakening needed to heal yourself, our population, and the planet.

My mission since I started my personal blog on DrLaurenCastle.com in 2019 has been, "Making health, well-being, and Functional Medicine affordable and accessible through the power of social media." It's been a journey as well to understand how I might make this happen, but I can look back now and see everything has come together to this point and see the potential for the future.

"Your training and preparation have brought you this far, but now the real healing begins, and it starts within you. Step into your power. Speak your truth. Live your life."

In Memory of Peggy Snell-Anderson: 11/10/1961-9/12/2021

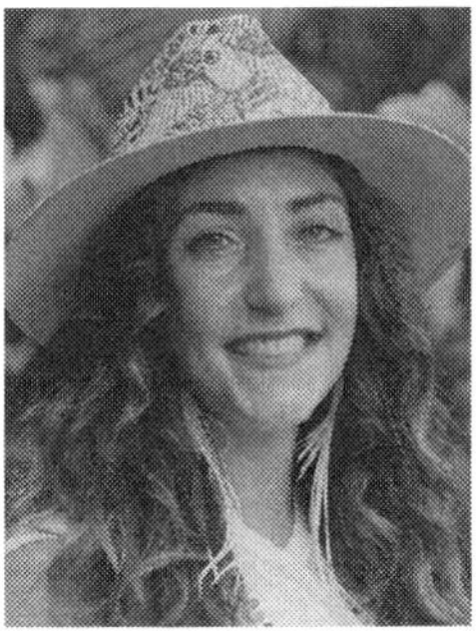

ABOUT DR. LAUREN CASTLE,

PHARMD, MS

Dr. Lauren Castle is the founder and CEO of the Functional Medicine Pharmacists Alliance, the first association representing pharmacists in functional medicine. FMPhA supports members practicing functional medicine across all pharmacy settings by uniting leaders in the field to provide continuing education, training, networking, and advocacy.

In addition to her role as CEO of FMPhA, is a functional medicine pharmacist with PharmToTable, and serves as secretary of the board for Con Smania Collective, a Transformational Retreat Center in Costa Rica.

Lauren received her Doctor of Pharmacy from Ohio Northern University in 2013 and her Master of Science in Human Nutrition and Functional Medicine from the University of Western States in 2018. Lauren has also studied with the Institute for Functional Medicine and the School of Applied Functional Medicine, becoming an Applied Functional Medicine Certified (AFMC) practitioner in 2022.

Lauren and her husband Seth live in Dayton, Ohio with their three cats, Olive, Pickle, and Fluffy. In their free time, you can find them riding motorcycles, attending music festivals, and exploring the world.

https://fmpha.org | https://drlaurencastle.com | https://consmaniacr.com

INFORMATION IS POWER

By: Dr. Anne Deukmedjian,
PHARMD, AFMCP, CSWWC, PLEI

"Listening is an act of love"
– Jim George

Imagine living every day as usual: functioning, working, and socializing normally. Nevertheless, after taking on a seemingly tame move to a new area, you develop sinus issues and a perpetual cough for months on end, with no relief despite taking rounds of different antibiotics. Symptoms progress, adding on bloody noses and then … HIVES! Gradually, the hives spread across your entire body, and you develop deep tissue swelling, called angioedema, which continuously travels to new areas of your body. While this is a difficult-to-imagine experience, after several healthy decades of life, I went through this exact scenario. How could the tables turn so quickly, from living healthily to living in a chronic, debilitating nightmare? Along with the unrelenting sinus issues, cough, nose bleeds, and hives came a rapid heartbeat, anxiety, brain fog, and headaches. My quality of life plummeted. I spent every second living within fully inflamed and uncontrollable skin, with no relief from medications and in too much discomfort to sleep. After months lacking clear cause or relief, I wondered if I'd have to live this way for the rest of my life.

Not wanting to face this fate, I resolved to find the answers. Over years on this quest, I depleted my entire health savings account making appointments with every specialist seeking answers. I saw an allergist/immunologist, a rheumatologist, an endocrinologist (two, actually), a couple of dermatologists, a gynecologist, a gastroenterologist, several primary care physicians, and urgent care and emergency room doctors. I became obsessed with learning anything and everything about hives and their triggers. I read studies, researched online, and investigated the ingredients in everything I consumed or applied to my skin. As a pharmacist myself, I also began researching every active and inactive ingredient in the medications I was taking against hives. Down the proverbial "rabbit hole" I went, searching for anything that would lead me toward resolution and healing.

Ever since I was born, it has been in my nature to ask "Why?", to seek deeper understandings, and to look beyond the surface. Now, the question for me to solve was, "What is happening to my body, and why is it so drastically off balance?" Unfortunately, the hives relentlessly continued with no relief, and almost every blood test came back "fine." I was eventually diagnosed with "chronic idiopathic urticaria," which meant that I had chronic hives with *unknown cause*. About six months of suffering with the hives, along with all the other symptoms, they suddenly stopped! Over the course of several more months, I slowly tapered off the plethora of medications I was taking, allowing my immune system to come back "online," and giving me the opportunity to perform allergy testing. I was apprehensive because the allergy tests could trigger my hives again, but I had to take the risk. I needed to know what my body was warning me against in order to ensure that it never happened again. We conducted every allergy skin prick test available without a single allergic response. My allergist/immunologist and I were both perplexed. Since I had a history of contact dermatitis, we also performed an array of skin patch chemical tests. I had many reactions to these, so, while I do not have allergies, I have confirmed chemical sensitivities.

I was so grateful for the relief that I moved forward, hoping my symptoms were just an abnormal one-off occurrence. Unfortunately, this was not the case. The hives returned in full force around the same month the following year. I thought to myself, "Oh, no ... here we go AGAIN?!?" I felt devastated. My allergist immediately put me back on the medications, attempting to stop my symptoms, but with no success. Since you can't be on high-dose prednisone long-term, I was presented with a new medication option to give me relief: an expensive monthly injectable immune modulator. I was caught between a rock and a hard place. Long-term intake of the oral medications I was currently taking wasn't an option, as continuous immune system suppression could cause some very serious health problems. Simultaneously, I couldn't stop the hives but did not want to use the monthly injectable. I didn't know if I would tolerate this new product, full of unfamiliar chemicals, slowly leaching into my body over the course of a month. This standstill was my turning point – the moment I realized that it was going to be up to me to discover my root cause. I did not want to cover up my issues with medications. I wanted to understand why so I could fix my problem from the source. I needed to find answers so I could live again, without medications, and to no longer feel beaten down and alone.

All my symptoms began after my relocation to this new city, an area that was exposed to a huge ongoing toxic natural gas and oil leak that made the news several years before my move. One night, as I scrolled through Facebook, I saw a post with pictures of a young woman with hives like mine. It was captioned: "The reaction my daughter got when she went back into the boxes stored in the basement from [the city I lived in]." I messaged the woman and shared that I was having the same problem while having gone to every specialist with no answers. She said that her daughter experienced the same scenario, and, after obtaining no answers or relief, they had to move elsewhere. Her daughter recovered after they moved. She informed me that I had likely been sensitized to one or more chemicals from the natural gas company operating locally. She advised me to move away from the area immediately, and that searching for answers with unaware medical professionals would be fruitless. The company was still actively using chemicals to pump, move, and store natural gas in the old petroleum oil holding tanks in the hills where I lived. Once again, I was told that my problem is chemicals.

Upon inquiring with the dermatologist I was seeing at the time, he confirmed what I already knew: any exposure via ingestion, absorption through skin, or inhalation can enter my bloodstream and cause a systemic reaction. This understanding and confirmation, along with depleting all other avenues, was enough for me to pack a backpack of essentials and immediately move to a hotel out of the area. While living in this hotel for a couple weeks, and implementing my new medically recommended diet, the itching in my lower legs slowly began to subside. Since I experienced some symptom improvement, I opted to live in different Airbnb's in a neighboring county for several months longer with my backpack of essentials. I was officially displaced from my home and all of my belongings, simply out of fear of exposure. When your health is on the brink and you know you can't live like this but also can't be on medications that will predispose you to bigger long-term problems, you make it happen, no matter the circumstances. If you don't have your health, you have nothing. So, I made it happen: hotels, Airbnbs, a backpack of essentials, clean water, clean skin products, and a gluten-free, anti-inflammatory, low-salicylate diet – all while living away from the supposed area of contamination where I became sick. I struggled with all these changes, but I slowly improved and was able to, once again, taper off my medications. I became well in this neighboring county, so I eventually rented an apartment there and started over from scratch.

All of this new information toward regaining my health brought up more questions: "Why did my reaction last for six months, stop for six months, and then begin again around the same time the next year?" The company was still operating around-the-clock after their monumental leak several years prior to my move. If this was the real cause of my problems, then how did I become hive-free while living there between my first and second episodes? I found another previous resident who was helping a local physician gather unbiased information regarding the effects of this multi-chemical leak on the community members. She shared that the timing of my hives made a lot of sense because the company restocked the pressurized holding tanks right before I was triggered both years. She further explained that, when tanks are restocked, the pressure increases within the tanks, and since they were old and not airtight, they released more chemicals during those months. More chemicals released means increased exposure and toxin body-burden during these months. Upon deeper contemplation and analysis, I acknowledged that I had several *non-symptomatic* family members living in this city. So, my next question to solve was: "Why are some locals struggling with these health symptoms while others are not?"

I may have won this battle but the war was not yet over. Despite improving and tapering off my hive medications, I would still periodically get flare-ups of fixed hives here and there. My issue was clearly not resolved, and I was terrified because since I did not know the exact cause of my issue, I did not know how to protect myself and prevent the hives from taking over. So, I rebuilt my empty apartment to be as clean and toxin-free as possible: an air purifier in every room, a water filtration system for my drinking water, clean skin products, a gluten-free diet, and a low salicylate diet upon any signs of flare-up. I became hyper-vigilant over the next few years, mentally logging all I was doing, eating, drinking, breathing, and putting on my skin. My goal was to become completely hive-free and no longer afraid of everything in life. I remember speaking to my dad, the person who knew me best in this world, and stating with resolve, "I won't stop until I find the cause," to which he paused, thought about it, and responded, "I know you will."

One day, I underwent a minor medical procedure with anesthesia and then immediately went to a week-long health retreat … and my hives resurfaced, as was usual during these years of my life. So, down the rabbit hole I go … researching again. This retreat was 100 percent plant-based, which helped me to realize that I needed the amino acids from animal protein to process chemicals out of my body. There it was: my lightbulb moment! *I am having a problem processing out various chemicals from my body!* My detoxification system was overtaxed and had reached a tipping point, pushing my body out of balance and into a highly reactive and inflamed state of being. This theory explains why some people reacted badly to the highly toxic area while others were fine: we all have different capacities for processing out toxins and chemicals from our bodies. This capacity is determined by various factors including nutrition, stress, and genetic predisposition. I had to ask myself … am I really the "Chemically Sensitive Pharmacist"?

It's ironic how life has a way of unfolding until you come full circle and find yourself staring straight at your life's purpose. I had to continue to understand my body and its limitations in our industrialized world, learn how to operate within these constraints, and use this knowledge to help myself and others. We are unnaturally bombarded with chemicals in our air, water, food, and skin. How do I live in a world full of chemicals when I have "chemical sensitivities"? How do I live healthily when my body is unable to release its chemical load as fast as it's being exposed to it? How do I fix this problem to avoid reaching my tipping point? Anesthesia, chemicals, toxins, natural gas, oil wells ... it's the chemicals. If this was my issue, then as an expert in this particular body process, I am the best equipped to solve my problem and regain my life. I felt hopeful again!

At this stage, I discovered Functional Medicine, which is defined by the Institute of Functional Medicine as a "systems biology-based approach that focuses on identifying and addressing the root cause of disease." I sought out a Functional Medicine provider to help me order laboratory tests not used in conventional medicine to assess body imbalance. Sure enough, we found that my body process dealing with removal of toxins and chemicals was operating sluggishly, leading to toxin overload. The labs also identified that I had been exposed to, and accumulated in my body, a petroleum-based toxin. My Functional Medicine provider used these results to determine which vitamins and supplements I needed to help support my sluggish body process and rebalance my system. Within two days, a fixed hive on my arm that I had been fearfully monitoring for months completely disappeared. My skin was free and clear of any evidence of systemic inflammation!

At this point, I was *sold* on Functional Medicine. My severe body imbalance, which stemmed from chemical sensitivities and systemic detoxification inefficiency coupled with the burden of chemical exposure, was solved with supplements and lifestyle changes! I didn't need to use medications to suppress my immune system and predispose me to other health issues later in life. I was so relieved to have obtained some answers, *but* I was also angry – angry that it took years of personal suffering to finally get to the bottom of it. I can't even imagine what my path would have looked like had I lacked my spirit, resolve, educational background, and resources to look beyond.

It became my mission to learn more, so I applied and was accepted into the Institute of Functional Medicine (IFM) Practitioner training program. It's an interesting world when we go back to the basics to learn advanced concepts and examine wellness from another perspective. My recovery and studies with IFM inspired me to open my own business where I could offer Functional Medicine support and resources to those seeking wellness from a different perspective. Therefore, I committed to the STORRIE Method group business development program to guide me in starting my business. The program was so helpful that I continued on to the STORRIE Institute™'s Wholistic Wellness Coaching™ certificate program afterwards. My goal was to provide individuals with a biology-based informational approach to learn about and optimize their own unique physiological system. At the pharmacy counter, patients approach me with these issues, while picking up medications for hives, chronic sinus issues, brain fog, headaches, lack of energy, or all kinds of sensitivities. Like me, these people need knowledge to support their path to wellness. It also became clear to me that, in our industrialized world, we are all overburdened and taxed with chemical stressors on our bodies, which can lead to chronic inflammation. Inflammation can, in turn, be the underlying culprit of many modern chronic health conditions. My life's purpose was unfolding through my own healing journey.

As I continued to study with the Institute of Functional Medicine, I conducted even more specialized laboratory tests on myself. Deeper down the rabbit hole I went, continuing on my journey of clarity and healing. I uncovered more answers, the most profound of which was my health genetic test revealing my specific genetic traits. This gave me the knowledge I needed to understand exactly where and how to support my system. We all have genetic traits that can be expressed when we are under stress: any and all systemic stressors can tip the scales of our bodies out of balance. Our tipping point and our traits are individually unique – no two people are exactly alike. Yet we all have the potential to lose balance and express these traits. The question is, do you know what your traits are and how to optimize your system to decrease the chance that they are ever expressed? I didn't, and I suffered because of it. Now, I know that I must focus on my lifestyle choices and keeping my body's toxic burden down. I also discovered that I have a genetic tendency to inefficiently process histamine (this is unsurprising, as histamine is also a chemical). Histamine is found in certain foods, wine, and bodily cells which initiate inflammatory responses. Looking back, I'm not surprised that my genetics test also pinpointed a caffeine sensitivity – another chemical. Having scientific, evidence-based confirmation was reassuring because I now knew exactly what to watch for instead of unknowingly fearing everything.

Our natural metabolic detoxification pathways include a process called biotransformation, in which a chemical compound undergoes biochemical modification to become a substance that can be eliminated successfully from our body. Chemicals may be derived from external, internal, synthetic, or environmental sources and require this detoxification process of biotransformation to convert substances into a form that can be released from our bodies. Biotransformation consists of two phases, phase I and phase II, that require certain vitamins and minerals for successful biochemical conversion of chemicals. When you have sluggish detoxification (like me), your phase II isn't able to keep up with your phase I detoxification process, producing accumulated toxic metabolites which cause oxidative stress, inflammation, and damage. It is important to ensure appropriately balanced detoxification in relation to our rate of exposure in order to maintain balance. I was inspired to call my business BioTransform, in recognition of my sluggish detoxification system that led me on my path to healing through Functional Medicine, and the resultant desire to help others with similar concerns. The name also denotes my desire to support those proactively seeking to optimize their own systems through a biological-based transformational wellness journey.

Looking back, I remembered that I had one random lip-swelling incident while in college. Doctors didn't find the cause and stated it was probably allergies. Now we know it was not allergies. During that episode, the doctors also found high bilirubin, a compound created internally during normal body processes, in my blood work. I was accordingly informed that I may have "Gilbert's Syndrome," which can cause accumulated bilirubin in the blood, and is considered harmless. This compound is large and needs to be properly broken down via the biotransformation detoxification process to be eliminated. I have since heard cutting-edge information from experts speculating that individuals with this condition should be monitored more closely, because if they have a problem eliminating this compound, they may also have issues with other large chemicals and hormone elimination that have to go through the same detoxification pathways to be eliminated from the body successfully. This potential accumulation of hormones and chemicals in the body, and resultant body imbalances, may predispose to develop other chronic conditions. Understanding my body with this new perspective shined a light on why I've also struggled with my hormones, such as debilitating menstrual cycle symptoms from my teenage years. Later in life, my endocrinologist and I spent years monitoring my slightly higher levels of another systemic hormone without explanation. It all makes sense once we acknowledge that hormones travel through the same biotransformation process as other large chemicals, such as bilirubin, to eliminate them from the body. If our body's process to remove these compounds is sluggish or inefficient, they will be out of balance and cause other systemic issues.

About a decade after my first lip swelling episode, I experienced another two random cases of lip swelling. I didn't know then what I know now, so I just attributed them to a supposed allergy to a new over-the-counter supplement I was taking both times from the same bottle. Now that I know I don't have allergies to this class of medication, or any other allergies, I suspect that the supplement had a chemical contamination in it, leading to a toxin exposure that caused the inflammatory swelling reactions. The veil of trust lifted, and I opened my eyes to the lack of purity, cleanliness, ingredient dosing accuracy, and effectiveness of supplements in the general marketplace. Many supplement companies do the bare minimum, using low quality or contaminated ingredients with no testing, simply to increase profits. Therefore, it is important to know and trust your supplement brands. If I have to take a supplement, it must be clean, safe, pure, and effective. Otherwise, I could amplify my problem and fall out of balance again. Ingesting any contaminants or simply not having the correct doses of vitamins or minerals will cause stress to my system and harm my health. I have since studied Functional Medicine supplement companies to choose the best for my system. Now, I am careful to recommend supplements from reputable sources where they openly test for quality ingredients that are clean and pure, contain correct dose amounts in the tablet, and are tested for clinical effectiveness. While these standards should be the baseline, they are, unfortunately, considered elite products today.

Several years after my first lip-swelling episode in college, I developed hypothyroidism like my mother and grandmother on my father's side. When I was diagnosed, it became my mission to learn as much as I could, and it's what motivated me to obtain my Doctorate of Pharmacy. It is well known that the thyroid is the first organ to be affected by environmental toxicity exposures. The medical community is also aware that patients with autoimmune thyroid issues, such as myself, have a higher risk of developing other autoimmune diseases over time. This potential autoimmune progression is inconsistent across individuals, and they don't know why it happens. I speculate, based on educated reasoning, that it is not the body itself predisposing these patients to progressively develop new autoimmune disorders, but rather it is the lack of toxin release. Over time, this uncorrected body inefficiency in an overburdened scenario leads to resultant inflammation and stress, progressively inflicting damage. In our current healthcare system, we use medications for symptom relief while leaving the core imbalance to potentially cause more damage over time. Sometimes, it's an even worse scenario when the medications for symptom control actually predispose you to other health issues. I'm not an extremist by any means, but I have to ask: Would this be an acceptable treatment plan for you as a patient?

Functional Medicine labs provided me with deep insights about my body to understand and support my unique system and its needs. Based on this information, I use air purifiers, live in a low-toxin area, drink filtered water, eat an organic diet that supports detoxification processes of the body, and take my trusted supplements. In fact, these lifestyle changes also alleviated my unusual joint inflammation and body aches. I am careful to limit my intake of gluten, histamine, caffeine, and salicylate rich foods. Now, I have nutriceuticals I can take that will help me break down some of these chemicals, if needed. I have been symptom-free for years since making these changes, and I am no longer afraid of everything in life. With the appropriate lifestyle adjustments for my specific system, I took back control and regained my life. As my book chapter title states: information is power!

Now that I was no longer in a crisis mode, I had time to reflect. I was so grateful for my extensive scientific background which spanned over two and a half decades, because I used it to regain my body balance and life back. Before obtaining my Doctorate of Pharmacy, I received my Bachelor's in Biological Sciences from the University of California, Irvine. Upon graduating with my Bachelor's degree, I taught science in the classroom, tutored advanced sciences, and worked at an outdoor science school as a naturalist. During my years working as a naturalist, I was the healthiest and happiest of my adult life. I lived in a community of like-minded colleagues, all together in one building in the middle of the forest. We took groups of kids out hiking and taught them about plants, animals, ecosystems, and the environment. I was at peace living in the middle of nature, far from the constant toxin exposure, and in the manner that human beings need to thrive: living with a socially connected community, hiking daily for movement, absorbing lots of sunlight, immersing in nature, eating healthy home cooked meals, and sleeping well. Unfortunately, our current standard of "normal" living isn't set up for our health and wellness. I experienced this gap upon leaving the outdoor science school and always yearned to go back to that lifestyle. Our supportive social community has been broken down in our current ways of living, and we, as human beings, have lost our sense of belonging, while being bombarded with too many unnatural chemicals, lack of nutrition and exercise, and insufficient sunlight or sleep. We are stressed on so many levels, and these stressors, over time, may trigger genetic trait expression. This is called epigenetics, which is the "study of how your behaviors and environment can cause changes that affect how your genes work" according to the Centers for Disease Control. This is a reversible phenomenon, making it evident that lifestyle and environmental factors are the baseline of health and wellness. The question now becomes, "How do we live in our current society and obtain all we need to thrive in optimal wellness without moving to a commune in the mountains?"

This is when I dove into my breathwork practice, as my health journey had taken its toll, and I wished to continue supporting my healing trajectory. I wanted to use all avenues to support toxin elimination, which occurs most optimally when in a rested state of body and mind, as well as through your lungs. Ironically, breathwork came into my life at the beginning of the COVID-19 pandemic in 2020, at the time when I was displaced from my home with hives and had moved to the new apartment in the neighboring county to start again. This apartment hired a breathwork instructor – now my breathwork instructor – to provide virtual breathing sessions during quarantine. My first session was powerful and transformative in a way words cannot describe.

Functional Medicine acknowledges that our entire physical system is affected by our emotional, mental, and spiritual bodies. They are interrelated, interconnected, and interdependent. As I practiced breathwork, I felt how connected my nervous system and well-being are, motivating me to utilize this modality as a complementary tool to support those seeking wellness. It was a blessing to be trained and obtain my advanced breathwork certification from BreatheOnIt® with Jay Bradley. I made new friends and explored new perspectives while learning this powerful modality based on yoga traditions. Breathwork benefits include inducing relaxation and happiness, decreasing negative feelings and body pains, increasing physical energy, boosting immunity, improving digestion and sleep, regulating blood sugar and pressure, releasing toxicity and trauma, opening energy centers to balance energy flow, and more. Breathwork allows us to regulate our nervous system, which supports our physical wellness, while elevating our consciousness to connect with source energy. I've had to ask myself: "What is our spiritual body exactly? How do we comprehend and explain that which we cannot see but can feel?" Everything we feel, whether it comes from physical, mental, emotional, or energetic sources, translates into resultant body chemistry, which affects us powerfully. This interconnectedness should be acknowledged, respected, and nurtured for our true holistic healing journey.

It was time for me to level up and support those seeking answers and information to optimize their personal wellness. My father lost his seven-year battle with cancer, and his brother also died from cancer at a very young age. I suspect that they may have had similar processing issues, like me. I won't ever be able to turn back time to know for sure or change the course of history. I wish that I could with every fiber of my being. Nevertheless, all I can do now is use my experience, information, and knowledge to support myself, my family, and all those who wish to lead their healthiest life. By doing so, I will know my life has a purpose and that my father's passing and my turbulent health journey have not been in vain.

As I envision my life's purpose and build upon these goals, I am excited to support those adults motivated to optimize their system for wellness in this overburdened, toxic world. I want to help people reclaim control over their lives using information, backed by science, while carefully listening to their bodies, minds, and souls. Further, while I traveled through my journey alone, it does not have to be that way for others: My dream is to create an interconnected community that supports internal self-exploration to enhance wellness. As author Jim George said, "Listening is an act of love," so let us listen to and learn about our system to make the appropriate adjustments that support us through our health transformation journeys.

Does my story resonate with you? Perhaps you, or someone you know, has been told you have high bilirubin or are sensitive to what seems like everything. Or maybe you have inexplicable sinus and pulmonary issues, fatigue, brain fog, insomnia, headaches, inflammation, weight issues, unexplained body aches, itching, history of hives, or "allergies" with no known conventional cause. Maybe you have ongoing thyroid and/or hormone imbalances that you have simply accepted as the norm in your life. Or perhaps you feel completely healthy and are simply interested in being proactive to learn about your personal system in a new way, and use this information to keep your body in tip-top shape as you move through life. At BioTransform LLC, we use various modalities to rebalance your nervous system while guiding energetic self-exploration and provide transformative holistic wellness coaching. Ultimately, we empower motivated adults with scientific information and supportive tools to function with renewed balance and vitality using specialized BioTransform™ health offers. If my story resonates with you, consider this as your invitation to connect and begin your transformative wellness journey!

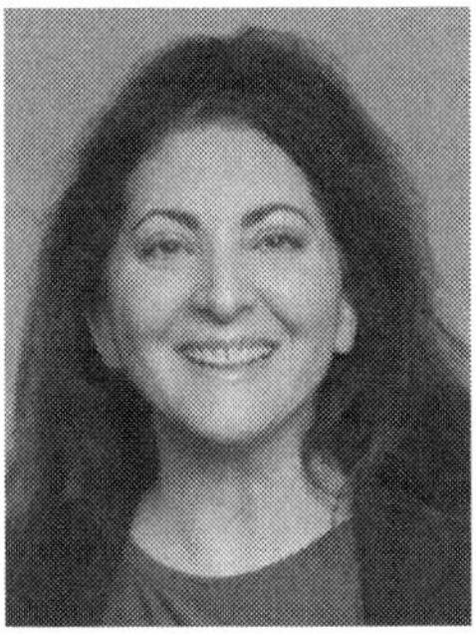

ABOUT DR. ANNE DEUKMEDJIAN,

PHARMD, AFMCP, CSWWC, PLEI

Dr. Anne is a board-licensed pharmacist, an advanced certified BreatheOnIt® Breathwork practitioner, and an Institute for Functional Medicine® practitioner candidate. She has an extensive scientific background spanning over two and a half decades which began when she earned her Bachelors in Biological Sciences from the University of California, Irvine. Prior to becoming a healthcare professional, Dr. Anne developed her scientific literacy and communication skills by working as a science teacher, an advanced sciences tutor, and a naturalist. She then earned her Doctorate of Pharmacy from Touro University, and has since practiced in community pharmacy for over 17 years, holding various leadership positions and obtaining multiple specialty certifications. Most recently, Dr. Anne is part of the 2023 graduating cohort at The Institute of Functional Medicine® upon completing the training "Applying Functional Medicine in Clinical Practice", and is continuing on to obtain her advanced practitioner certificate training. She is also currently in the process of becoming a Certified STORRIE Wholistic Wellness Coach™ (CSWWC) from STORRIE Institute™.

Dr. Anne was inspired to build her business, BioTransform™ LLC, after experiencing her own personal health crisis, from which she found eventual relief and a wellness transformation by harnessing functional medicine and breathwork. She draws upon her deep education, breadth of experiences, natural analytical skills, and energetic connectivity to support clients through their wellness journeys. Dr. Anne is both personally and professionally interested in the topic of overcoming environmental, chemical, metabolic, and energetic stressors using breathwork, epigenetic modifications, and biohacking to restore and maintain internal body balance.

Dr. Anne empowers motivated adults with scientific information and supportive tools to function with renewed balance and vitality using specialized BioTransform™ health offerings.

www.DrAnneDeukmedjian.com | www.BioTransformHealth.com
Dr.Anne@BioTransformHealth.com | IG: @BioTransformHealth

FROM PHARMACY TO WHOLISTIC WELLNESS: A GREEK JOURNEY OF FAMILY, FOOD AND HEALING

Dr. Georgianne Douglas,
PHARMD, CSWWC

"Let food be thy medicine and medicine be thy food."

– Hippocrates

Transform your health and reclaim your vitality with Dr. Georgianne Douglas, the Mediterranean Health Coach, who empowers busy professionals and parents to effortlessly embrace the Mediterranean lifestyle for longevity and quality of life.

Growing up in a traditional Greek family, I had the fortune of seeing delicious and healthy Mediterranean food served at almost every meal as a child. I knew that home-cooked meals and eating together with siblings, parents, and grandparents was a special thing that my family emphasized, but it wasn't until much later that I realized that this lifestyle was also the reason for longevity and quality of life free from chronic disease. Even after pharmacy school and years of counseling patients in a community pharmacy setting, and seeing the limitations of conventional medicine in treating chronic illnesses by merely addressing symptoms without addressing the underlying causes, I still didn't understand the true connection of "food as medicine." I finally understood once I began to educate myself on the wonderfully simple concept of Functional Medicine and treating the body as a whole, from inside out, by uncovering the root cause. This Wholistic Wellness approach resonated deeply with me as a Greek-food-loving naturalist, and the key feature of biochemical individuality taught in Function Medicine resonated with me as a pharmacist and healthcare professional. The discovery was so powerful that it has led me to leave my traditional role as a well-compensated, full-time dispensing pharmacist. I decided to take action through passion-driven work and create a Mediterranean Health Coaching service that helps clients improve health outcomes with chronic disease through an emphasis on fresh vegetables and fruit, whole grains, legumes, olive oil and fish – just like my Greek ancestors and the traditional food cultures of countries that surround the Mediterranean Sea.

This journey from pharmacist to health and wellness coach instilled in me a recognition of the power of a Wholistic Wellness approach, which encompasses not only physical health but also mental, emotional, and spiritual well-being.Being a Wholistic Wellness practitioner means adopting a comprehensive and integrative approach to health and healing. It involves recognizing that human beings are complex systems with interconnected aspects, and that to achieve true well-being, all of these aspects must be considered. Wholistic Wellness practitioners see individuals as unique, understanding that each person's body, mind, and spirit interact in a highly individualized manner. In my case, it means utilizing my background as a pharmacist and healthcare professional, along with my passion for Greek cuisine and Mediterranean food culture, to empower and educate my clients on the benefits of adopting a Wholistic Wellness lifestyle.

My upbringing in a large and close-knit family was marked by a deep connection to our Greek heritage, instilled by my parents, who immigrated to America in their youth, seeking a new beginning and brighter prospects for their children. My grandparents, who lived with us, served as a living link to our culture, language, and traditional cuisine from the old country. The vibrant memories of our family dinners, where kids, parents, and grandparents gathered almost every night, remain etched in my heart.

In our home, mindful eating was a way of life. During the warm summers, our garden provided us with fresh produce, inspiring the creation of home-cooked meals that embraced the changing seasons. We never had a summer without cucumbers, tomatoes, and oregano, the key ingredients in our staple Classic Greek Village Salad (Horiatiki). We ate vegetables, fresh herbs, and fish often, while meat was consumed sparingly, and desserts were reserved for joyous occasions and holidays, heightening the sense of togetherness and celebration.

What made our family's story even more remarkable was the longevity and vitality of my grandparents. Even into their 90s, they remained actively engaged in life, tending to their garden and taking regular evening walks. Their commitment to a lifestyle rich in seasonal food was evident as they gathered with us to prepare meals, their hands skillfully cleaning and chopping vegetables for our family gatherings.

My parents have emulated their example, and now in their 70s, they enjoy good health without relying on any medication or battling chronic illnesses.

Beyond their culinary practices, my parents and grandparents led a spiritually fulfilling life. They balanced their work commitments with active involvement in the church community, and volunteered at cultural festivals and events, fostering a sense of purpose and connection.

Reflecting on their choices and lifestyle, I now realize that my ancestors were, unknowingly, pioneers of what we now call lifestyle medicine. They embodied the key principles of the Mediterranean diet: embracing variety, moderation, and the predominance of vegetables over animal-sourced foods. Their lives were a testament to a philosophy that cherished personal relationships, the pursuit of happiness, and the value of physical activity.

As I progressed through pharmacy school and entered the Western healthcare field, I encountered numerous patients struggling with chronic diseases like hypertension, diabetes, and hyperlipidemia. It became evident that many of them lacked the foundation of sound nutrition from childhood, making it challenging for them to adopt healthy lifestyle changes in adulthood once the diseases had already taken hold. I felt a deep sense of empathy for these individuals and a desire to find a solution that addressed the root cause of their health issues.

It was during this time, through my personal development journey, deeply involved in listening to alternative healthcare and entrepreneur podcasts, that I was introduced to Functional Medicine – a paradigm that resonated deeply with me. The idea of using food as medicine and focusing on addressing the underlying imbalances within the body struck me as intuitive and powerful. I realized that Functional Medicine was the missing link in my pharmacy education, providing me with the tools and knowledge to counsel patients on implementing practical and sustainable changes to their diet and exercise routines.

Drawing on my Greek heritage and passion for Mediterranean cuisine, I discovered a unique way to merge my background as a pharmacist with my love for wholesome food culture. By combining my experience growing up in a kitchen with three generations of Greek women with the principles of Functional Medicine, I found the perfect fit for my path as a Wholistic Wellness practitioner. As a Mediterranean Health Coach, I can empower and educate clients on the benefits of adopting a Wholistic Wellness lifestyle.

In my professional role as a Mediterranean Health Coach, I leverage my pharmacy experience and healthcare expertise to guide clients toward healthier choices in both nutrition and lifestyle. By incorporating the wisdom of the Mediterranean diet and Functional Medicine principles, I help individuals identify and address the root causes of their health challenges, offering personalized strategies to promote well-being from the inside out.

Through my coaching, clients learn to embrace the Mediterranean philosophy of balanced nutrition, physical activity, and the nurturing of meaningful relationships. I firmly believe that small, consistent changes can lead to transformative outcomes, and my mission is to support and empower my clients on their journey to improved health and vitality.

As a passionate advocate for Wholistic Wellness, I am dedicated to bridging the gap between traditional healthcare and lifestyle medicine. By fusing my professional background with the richness of Mediterranean food culture, I aim to inspire a new generation to embrace a lifestyle that nourishes the body, mind, and spirit, unlocking the full potential of human health and happiness.

It is my belief that our healthcare systems often focus more on treating diseases after they have already developed rather than emphasizing preventive care. It's a truth we recognize – a drug that's curative for one can be perilous for another. Our tendency to heavily rely on pharmaceutical interventions can yield unintended harm. Instinctively, we anticipate a uniform response to a specific drug among patients. Yet, we overlook the reality that individuals possess varying levels of receptors for each drug, precluding a standardized reaction. The inclination is to introduce new medications to an existing regimen when response is inadequate. We may occasionally attribute insufficient drug adherence to patients, yet the issue might stem from excessive prescribing. These gaps are substantial, and they open the door for Wholistic Wellness practitioners to offer meaningful contributions. Here are some of those gaps and how Wholistic Wellness practitioners can contribute:

- **Preventive Care:** Healthcare systems often focus on treating diseases after they have already developed rather than emphasizing preventive care. A Mediterranean Health Coach can promote preventive measures through education, lifestyle modifications, and personalized diet plans based on the Mediterranean diet, which has been associated with various health benefits like the reduction in inflammation, cardiovascular risk, and overall mortality.
- **Chronic Disease Management:** Chronic diseases like obesity, diabetes, and cardiovascular conditions are becoming increasingly prevalent and costly to manage. This topic resonates with me as I have personal experience working as a Clinical Consultant Pharmacist in a primary care private practice setting before I found my niche as a Mediterranean Health Coach. As a Clinical Consultant, I implemented a chronic care management program in an urban, low-income community in East Charlotte, North Carolina, serving some of the sickest ambulatory care patients who struggled with access to healthcare. I found that I had the greatest

impact on improving health outcomes through the monthly check-ins and preventative health conversations I carried out with my patients. However, the limitations and red tape around complicated and confusing billing codes for government insurance reimbursement was what led me to find a way to practice chronic disease management through Functional Medicine and Wholistic Health Coaching that bypasses all insurance parameters all together. Functional Medicine aims to address the root causes of these diseases rather than just managing symptoms. A health coach can work with patients to identify triggers, implement lifestyle changes, and encourage compliance with treatment plans. And when this is done with patient-centered health goal setting, the greatest results can be achieved.

- **Patient Education and Empowerment:** Many patients lack sufficient knowledge about their health conditions and the potential impact of lifestyle choices. A health coach can act as an educator, helping patients understand the importance of nutrition, exercise, stress management, and sleep in achieving overall well-being. In this generation of social media and artificial intelligence, anyone can conduct their own research on their current health issue. The problem is not how to find an answer, but rather how to discern what information to believe amid the plethora of search results. This is where a health coach can be the perfect sounding board to lean on as an adjunct to one's existing traditional healthcare providers.
- **Lifestyle Medicine Integration:** Healthcare systems often struggle to integrate lifestyle medicine into traditional care models. According to American College of Lifestyle Medicine, the six pillars of lifestyle medicine are whole-food, plant-predominant eating

patterns; physical activity; restorative sleep; stress management; avoidance of risky substances; and positive social connections. A Mediterranean Health Coach can serve as a bridge, collaborating with medical professionals to complement treatment plans with lifestyle interventions and personalized diet plans based on the Mediterranean diet

- **Mental Health Support:** Mental health issues are on the rise, and there is a need for more comprehensive support beyond medication and therapy alone. A Wholistic Wellness approach can encompass mental well-being, encouraging practices like mindfulness, meditation, and emotional self-care. Reflecting on my personal voyage of career transition, navigating the challenges of working in retail pharmacy amidst the worldwide COVID-19 pandemic, and managing the responsibilities of raising two kids under the age of two while sustaining a full-time job and establishing a consulting enterprise, I discovered that practices like yoga, meditation, and regular outdoor walks were instrumental in maintaining my equilibrium.
- **Cultural Sensitivity:** Traditional healthcare systems may not always fully understand or account for cultural differences in diet and lifestyle practices. A Mediterranean Health Coach, who is familiar with the cultural nuances of the region, can provide more tailored and culturally sensitive advice to individuals who are busy with their careers and their families. For example, as a pharmacist working in a community setting, serving patients on a daily basis with my Spanish and Greek language skills, I saw first-hand the impact language has on clear communication, building trust and rapport, cultural sensitivity, reduced anxiety, and avoiding medication errors. Overall, speaking the patient's native language

is a crucial aspect of providing patient-centered care. It enhances communication, and promotes patient engagement, ultimately leading to better health outcomes and overall satisfaction with healthcare services.

- **Nutrition and Dietary Guidance:** Nutrition plays a crucial role in health, and the Mediterranean diet is well-regarded for its cardiovascular and anti-inflammatory health benefits. A health coach can provide personalized dietary guidance based on an individual's health status, preferences, and lifestyle, helping patients adopt healthier eating habits. In the words of the ancient Greek physician, Hippocrates, "If we could give every individual the right amount of nourishment and exercise, not too little and not too much, we would have found the safest way to health."
- **Lifestyle Modifications:** Many health issues are aggravated by poor lifestyle choices such as sedentary behavior, smoking, and excessive alcohol consumption. As a food-loving Greek pharmacist passionate about healthy eating, when I think about the Mediterranean way of eating, I look at it as a lifestyle. It's not so much what we eat, which is beneficial and anti-inflammatory; it's in how we eat it. We eat with enjoyment and *orexi* (the Greek word for good appetite). We eat with loved ones. A Mediterranean Health Coach can assist individuals in making sustainable lifestyle modifications, encouraging physical activity, stress reduction, and healthy habits.

By incorporating Functional Medicine and Wholistic Wellness principles, a Mediterranean Health Coach can contribute to filling these gaps in the healthcare system. However, it's essential to note that health coaches' roles complement but do not replace that of doctors or other healthcare providers. Collaborative efforts between health coaches and healthcare professionals are crucial for delivering comprehensive and effective patient care.

Embrace the beauty of preventative lifestyle habits, drawing inspiration from the relaxed Mediterranean way of life. Prioritize humility, cherishing family first, and savor the abundance of wholesome foods, nourishing your body and soul with the essence of the Mediterranean diet. Cultivate a relaxed and harmonious approach to well-being, where the joy of simple pleasures and meaningful connections lay the foundation for a vibrant and fulfilling life.

- Supporting Facts, Research, Content
    - The Institute For Functional Medicine (https://www.ifm.org/functional-medicine/)
    - Diet Review: Mediterranean Diet | The Nutrition Source by Harvard University (https://www.hsph.harvard.edu/)
    - Dr. Georgianne Douglas—Functional Medicine Health Coach—GD Pharmacy Consulting, LLC (www.drgeorgiannedouglas.com)
    - Article from Open Access Pub - Culture and Mediterranean Diet by Iglesias López | 1Universidad Francisco de Vitoria, Faculty of Health Sciences, Spain
    - Article from National Institutes of Health, National Library of Medicine, "Are we over-dependent on pharmacotherapy?" https://www.ncbi.nlm.nih.gov/pmc/articles/PMC2745859/
    - American College of Lifestyle Medicine https://lifestylemedicine.org

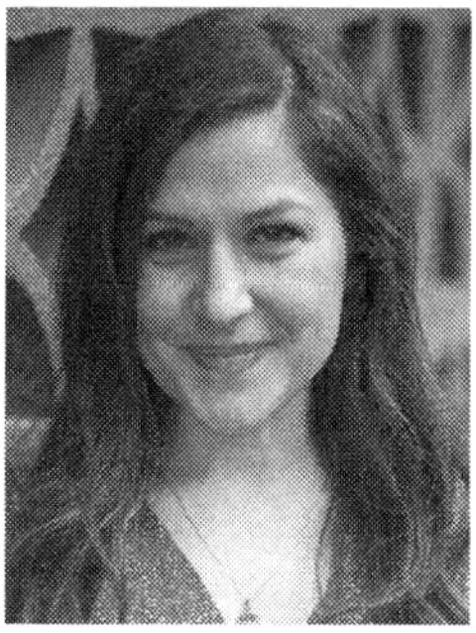

ABOUT DR. GEORGIANNE DOUGLAS,

PHARMD, CSWWC

Dr. Georgianne Douglas is a pharmacist turned Mediterranean Health Coach, Wholistic Wellness Practitioner, and speaker. She hosts a recurring Mediterranean Cooking Demo where she has been recognized for her voice in addressing the gaps in healthcare through the practice of functional medicine. She helps busy professionals & parents go from feeling stressed about their health challenges to effortlessly making healthy food & lifestyle choices. With her proprietary Mediterranean-style strategies, you can now use food as medicine and transform your eating habits. Her focus on the Mediterranean diet is deeply intertwined with her Greek family heritage.

As the Founder and CEO of GD Pharmacy Consulting, LLC Dr. Georgianne is bridging the gap in healthcare between preventative medicine and chronic disease management. After spending more than a decade seeing patients in her pharmacy practice continue to decline in health as the healthcare system led them down the path of "a pill for every ill", Dr. Georgianne discovered a new passion in life in teaching people about how healthy eating habits can transform our lives not only for longevity, but also quality.

Through her experience counseling patients on health challenges like hypertension, diabetes and high cholesterol, she has seen first hand the struggle to implement lifestyle changes that we all know are good for us. With life lessons from 3 generations of Greek women before her, and years of travel through Mediterranean countries like Greece, Italy, Spain, France, Croatia, Turkey and Egypt, she has used these experiences to create a framework for helping clients optimize their health and reduce chronic disease through her easy to implement strategies.

She is a frequent speaker on holistic healing from the inside out, preventative health benefits of the Mediterranean way of eating, gut-skin health connections, and fertility + Mediterranean Diet. She has spoken on podcasts like WSIC "The L Show", STORRIE™ Podcast, and "Rising into Mindful Motherhood" Podcast. Dr. Georgianne is currently enrolled in STORRIE Institute™ to become a Certified STORRIE Wholistic Wellness Coach™ (CSWWC).

Dr. Georgianne believes that drawing on the inspiration from the relaxed Mediterranean way of life, we can all learn to cherish family first, and savor the abundance of wholesome foods to nourish and heal our body and soul from the inside out.

www.drgeorgiannedouglas.com | info@drgeoriganne douglas.com |
IG: @drgeorgiannedouglas

FROM CHRONIC DIETING TO WHOLE-BODY *WELLNESS*

By: Tara Durden,
MS, RDN

"When you up-level your idea of what's possible, and decide to really go for it, you open yourself up to the means to accomplish it as well."

– Jen Sincero, Author of "You are a Badass"

I thought I was going to diet forever. Until my spirit and metabolism crashed.

I was fatigued, my weight had plateaued, and I couldn't have been more confused. Wasn't I supposed to feel great? I was doing everything you're supposed to. I had rid my home and body of everything "bad," and I was doing what the experts recommended. "Work out this much." "Only eat these foods in this way." "Do this and you'll look and feel like me." How could I have possibly messed this up? It was through this difficult time that I learned this in fact was not a sustainable way of living.

Decades later, the power of holistic healing and Functional Medicine opened my eyes, opened my eyes so wide that I couldn't help but delve deeper. Since wellness was a keen interest of mine, I wanted to learn more. What I once thought was "wellness" shifted to a totally different perspective – to my definition of wellness today. I underestimated the power of whole-body wellness, from the inside out. And that is what I love most about Functional Medicine, the ability to heal from the inside out.

Growing up, I was surrounded by a family who loves food. My grandma, mom, and aunt were always in the kitchen cooking and baking. Food was our love language, a way to gather and a way to celebrate life. My grandmother was also in the field of nutrition, and hosted her own cooking show called *Naomi's Kitchen*.

Starting in kindergarten, cheerleading became my hobby. I cheered through eighth grade. Then, I swam for the high school swim team for three years. There were guidelines about what and how to eat, but I didn't understand macronutrients or how to balance meals. Since I was the teen who carried some extra weight, I was very self conscious. Diet culture never failed to encourage me to try to look a certain way, to fit society's standards. Once I was able to make the conscious decision to diet, you bet I jumped on that train. Because my mom's generation was a time of Atkins and Weight Watchers, I was first-handedly exposed. Early on, I experimented with crash dieting, counting calories, and exchanging exercise for food (a big OUCH to your metabolism!). I thought this was the way to do it – the experts said so. I soon realized (the not-so-fun way) the damage I was doing to my metabolism, hormones, and overall health. It was a constant, exhausting battle trying to diet and exercise enough to keep the weight off. Once I got to college, the free gym was my outlet to burn calories. I thought about how perfect it would be to do cardio for hours. I'd go back to my dorm room mini fridge and opt for the lowest calorie option to eat after my workout. Of course that was likely something with little to no protein. No wonder I was starving and unable to get quality sleep through the night.

Research shows that we don't fail diets – diets fail us. I'm intuitive, yet I ignored my gut feeling that dieting couldn't be a sustainable way to live. Over my course of chronic dieting, my metabolism gradually started adapting to fewer calories. This made it extremely difficult to continue to lose weight, at least safely.

Becoming a nutritionist didn't cross my mind until my 20s. I dreamt of becoming a speech-language pathologist. That dream soon came to an end after years of schooling and an internship that finalized my decision. This was *not* my dream – it didn't fulfill my adult self any longer. I knew I was put on this Earth to be a "helper," but it wasn't this. My husband and I floated some ideas around since I was close to graduation without a plan. Nutrition popped up. I'd always loved being active and I loved food. A month post-graduation, I was back in school giving the basic courses of nutrition a go. This felt more aligned. The deeper I dug into the field, the more I could relate to how nutrition works synergistically with the body. I realized that dieting was not a priority, but having a positive relationship with food and myself *was*. Being able to learn about the body through science was intriguing. After relearning hunger cues (which took loads of time and conditioning since I'd ignored them for years), getting to know who I was and wanted to be, becoming more mindful, balancing my plate, and working out for enjoyment versus punishment, I knew this was the career I'd like to pursue.

Getting my second bachelor's degree was on the simpler side since I had the basics done from my first degree. Well, it may not have been easy but it was definitely quick. To become a Registered Dietitian-Nutritionist, you require a master's degree along with 1200 hours of supervised practice (in the hospital, skilled nursing facility, and community settings) prior to sitting for the national credentialing exam. Not to mention, the internships push that these three settings are the best career options out there for dietitians. During my clinical hospital rotation, I loved how busy I was, though I was extremely nervous to start since I never felt comfortable in hospitals. I was on the go, always learning something new and collaborating with the entire interdisciplinary team. At this point, I thought "this could be it," my forever career. I continued dedicating all of my time to finishing my graduate courses, doing my unpaid supervised practice hours, and attempting to work part time (hello burnout). This was a stressful time in my life, but now that I look back on it, it was worth it. Just as I was sitting for the national exam, the pandemic hit. There was such uncertainty in the world. Everything shut down, but I was still able to work remotely with the pediatric outpatient clinic (that was my community rotation, and they ended up hiring me). I had extra time on my hands, lots of it (who didn't?). I started to dabble in the world of social media from a dietitian's perspective. I featured cooking demos and random recipes and never thought anything of it. It turned into my creative outlet.

Once the pandemic slowed, I left the clinic and accepted two new part-time positions, one at a hospital and another at a skilled nursing home. The more I counseled patients, the more I felt misaligned. I didn't like how short my interactions were with patients, counseling them and then leaving them on their own to get discharged. I didn't get to know them or build a relationship with them. I longed for more as a dietitian. I wanted to see their wellness journeys and how they progressed.

The more I used Instagram, the more I connected with women who were similar to the woman I once was, dieting, with a poor relationship with food and their bodies. I thought this may be an opportunity to help them. I felt like entrepreneurship was in my blood, especially because my dad is an entrepreneur. I was under the impression that starting a practice required years of experience at a hospital or a skilled nursing home, so I continued working at both. I thought, why not start a little nutrition coaching "side hustle." And that's when my company was born.

In the beginning, my mission was to help women and men overcome dieting and learn about whole-body wellness. Instead of taking away from the body, it was important to learn how to give back to the body. The more women I helped, the more hormone and gut health issues became apparent. Almost all of the women I was helping were currently taking some form of birth control, or had in the past. This was an ah-ha moment. These were the exact shoes I was in. I took birth control for almost two decades, and during the majority of that time, I was dieting. It wasn't until switching providers that I learned oral contraceptives were actually *not* helping my situation. Being on birth control for over a decade deteriorated my overall health. My new provider encouraged me to ditch the pill, use FAM (fertility awareness method), and check the health of my hormones in the event that I did become pregnant. To this day, I have so much respect for my new provider. When a provider dismisses symptoms (ruptured cysts, heavy, painful, and irregular periods) and doesn't look into the root of it potentially relating to hormonal birth control, RUN! My hormone and stool test results showed very low sex hormones, whacky cortisol patterns, and overgrowth of bad gut bugs. My Functional Medicine practitioner crafted some gut and hormone healing protocols for me. I began healing from the inside out. My energy came back, my belly was feeling better, I rarely bloated after meals, and my sleep quality improved. I saw the power that Functional Medicine held, and that's when my company started evolving even further.

Labs interested me from the get-go. I like numbers, and both of my parents are in the accounting field. When I came across the opportunity to learn more about functional labs through a dietitian-led program, I was hooked. The program focused on extensive blood labs, hormone panels, stool-testing panels, and vitamin and mineral panels. Since I was transitioning off the pill and healing my hormones at this same time, it was fitting. This would be an awesome opportunity to continue to learn more to help others going through a similar situation.

Since becoming an advanced lab testing practitioner, I've been helping women balance hormones and heal digestive issues using functional and sustainable methods. My clients often come to me when they're looking for more than what their primary care providers can offer. My practice is very unique and individualized. I am all ears prior to creating their customized health plan. My goal is for clients to feel nourished and confident in their bodies again. Setting them up to be nourished enough for preconception, regardless of whether they are actively trying to conceive or not, is a big deal. In my case, I was in my healing journey and got pregnant unexpectedly. I always knew I wanted to be a mom at some point, but my husband and I weren't in that season of life yet – we were traveling and working hard! The overwhelm soon became excitement. Ironically enough, my practice was starting to pick up. More and more women who were new moms or moms with major gut and hormonal imbalances were seeking my services. What good timing.

I'm going on my third year practicing with Functional Medicine and it just keeps getting better. Nutrition and Functional Medicine are young sciences, so it's amazing to see new studies and research coming out left and right. I'm constantly learning new trends, myths, and protocols to ensure my clients get the care they deserve. Women finish their time with me with not only improved gut and hormone health but also a positive mindset around food and themselves.

My holistic wellness practice has evolved quite a bit from what it started as. I don't just teach women how to eat. In fact, that's only a fraction of what we touch on for the duration of working together. I use a nourishment fundamental baseline that consists of topics such as nutrition, movement, self-care, hydration, gut health, and sleep hygiene. Prior to any functional testing and supplements, I encourage clients to get their bodies ready for healing. Ensuring they are eating balanced meals, working to balance their blood sugar, minimizing stress, creating mindfulness, optimizing their nervous system, and sleeping enough are some ways to prepare. These are habits I've carried over into my daily routine. When I'm overwhelmed, I like to come back to my "why" and stand by these practices. I hope that you too can find daily habits that you enjoy and carry out throughout your wellness journey. There is no better time than now to get started!

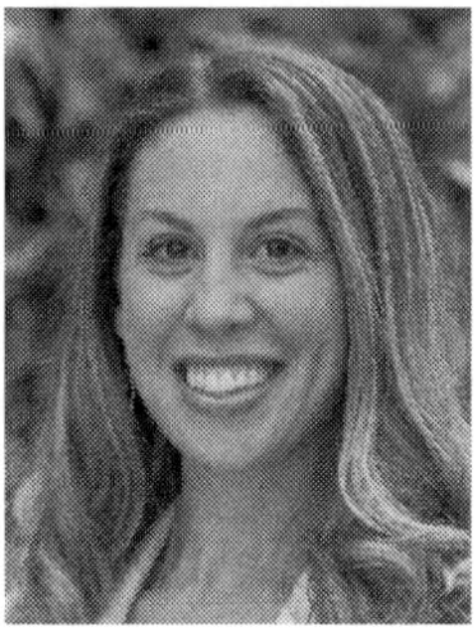

ABOUT TARA DURDEN,

MS, RDN

Tara Durden is a Functional Registered Dietitian-Nutritionist specializing in women's health. She has worked with women all over the country struggling with hormonal and digestive issues using a functional and sustainable approach to optimize overall health and well-being.

Her passion for helping others started out as a dream to become a Speech Pathologist but she realized that was not her forte. The universe had other plans for her and that's when nutrition surfaced. After obtaining her first Bachelor's degree, she found herself back in school and achieved her Bachelor of Science degree in Nutrition and Master of Science in Nutrition soon after.

For the past decade, she has worked in multiple healthcare settings including outpatient clinics, hospitals, long term care and private practice. Her role as a dietitian has been to provide the best plan of care and most sustainable wellness plan for patients and clients. When corporate medical settings no longer served her, she followed solely down the path of private practice and that's when her company was born.

Drawing from her personal wellness endeavors and professional experiences, she has learned that to achieve the optimal wellness she always sought, a personalized and holistic approach is required. Using a functional nutrition approach, Tara was able to optimize her hormones and gut health. Now feeling the best in her body that she ever has (even after becoming a mama with another on the way), she is passionate about helping you feel the same. Today, she helps women like you optimize hormones, mineral status and gut health combining both holistic and scientific methods. She guides and supports you during your whole body healing journey.

www.nutrition-thyme.com | tarathedietitian@gmail.com |
IG: @nutritionwithtara_

THE JOURNEY OF "SUCCESS" TO SERENITY

By: Casey Fisk,
CSWWC

"Alone we can leave an impression, together we can change the world. Let's join together and embrace the gifts that God has given us on this earth, share them with as many people as we possibly can, so that we all may bless others in this beautiful life."

– Casey Fisk

I had it all. Or so it seemed. I had the beautiful home on the water, the nice car, the fancy corporate job, not a worry in the world about money, abundant vacations, full flexibility in my schedule, the ability to work from home when I wanted, a family full of love and support, a spouse who I am madly in love with and supports me, and most importantly, the good health of my son and husband. Then why did I feel so empty?

I felt guilty for feeling empty, which then made it even worse. I knew that there were so many people praying for what I already had, so why did I not enjoy it to its full potential? Why did I feel numb all the time? Why couldn't I quiet the constant to-do list in my mind and enjoy the present moment? What was wrong with me? Why did I constantly feel like something was missing or I wasn't doing something right? Why did my physical body feel so bad and have multiplying negative symptoms? Why did I have constant anxiety to the point of jaw-shaking panic attacks?

My mind couldn't stop. I was always on the go right up until I crashed at night, just to wake up and do it all again. And again. And again. But that's why I was "successful," right? I couldn't slow down. No way! I had to provide, I had things to do, money to make, people to answer to, a family to take care of, and so I just had to keep pushing myself. If I am not going to do it, then who will, right?

That was my mindset. Every day.

My breaking point came when one day I had back-to-back calls all day. On the phone I was great, but between calls I literally felt the sensation of choking, followed by sets of full-blown panic attacks. This was the way I had been functioning, and it was unfortunately becoming my "norm." A huge part of my high-pressure job was to put a smile on and encourage people to take a leap of faith, let go of fear, and move forward with their goals. All the while, I felt like I had a brewing volcano inside my mind and body that was about to erupt at any given moment.

My husband walked in with a glass of wine … at 2 p.m. … on a workday. He was trying to convince me to drink it to calm down. From the outside he saw me spiraling, and he didn't know how else to calm my mind down. That hit me like a ton of bricks. That was the first (and last) time that happened. Something had to change, and quickly.

What led me here? Well, let's back up to several key phases in my life that piled on top of one another, which ultimately spiraled me down into this valley I was currently in.

Stress was always a component of my life, as is the case for most Americans these days. I was never really taught ways to handle stress other than to be told, "You have to relax." I would think, "Uhhh, relax? What does that even mean, and who has the time to do that anyways?" From the time I was a child, I was that type A, go-getter, work-your-ass-off kinda gal. When I was 14, I started working 10-hour days on the weekends cleaning beach condos. From there, as soon as I was "officially" allowed to work, I had at least two jobs at a time until after my son was born. At that point, I traded in the second job for being a mom and to focus on climbing the corporate ladder as fast as I could. Stress, stress, and more stress, without a release.

When my son was 6 months old, I got that dreaded phone call that no one ever wants to receive: "Your dad has terminal cancer, and they say he has less than a year to live. You probably want to get here as quickly as you can." Against all odds, that determined man persevered for 10 beautiful years full of amazing memories and precious moments. He never EVER complained, regardless of the massive amount of pain he was in every day. He taught our family an extremely powerful lesson: Strength and healing comes from your mind and your perspective. He utilized the power of his mind to overcome so many obstacles all the way up until his time on Earth was done. I was a daddy's girl, so of course his passing had a very troubling effect on me. As time has continued on and my mind has begun to clear, I can reflect more and more on the lessons he taught everyone around him and understand the true power he held. He knew his strength came from God, and he knew his power came from his mind. He didn't know how to be negative or to have "bad energy." All he knew was to live each precious moment with endurance and control of his mind. This planted a seed in me that I later was able to start harnessing myself. When I held his hand as he left this world and entered his heavenly home, I believe his strength and perseverance infused into my soul. As hard as that moment in time was, it was beautiful at the same time.

In the meantime, the volcano inside me continued to fizzle up since I did not understand the importance at that time of releasing emotions and stress. It started to manifest in my body as a multitude of extreme physical symptoms. I spent a lot of time (and thousands of dollars) going to specialist after specialist, just to be told "I don't know why you have all these symptoms – it all looks good on your test and bloodwork, but take this prescription and it should help alleviate some of the symptoms you are experiencing. Oh, and maybe you should see a psychiatrist too." I knew something was not right in my body. How could I be having all of these rashes, swelling, daily debilitating migraines, constant weight gain, dizziness, blurry vision, hair loss, low heart rate, bloating, memory problems, fatigue, and anxiety and extreme panic if nothing was "physically wrong with me"?

My next stop was to the allergist. Once I had my allergy test done, I figured out I was pretty much allergic to everything. The allergist told me that the only way to stay away from everything I am allergic to is to "wear white gloves like Minnie Mouse and put myself in a plastic bubble." Clearly I wasn't going to be able (or willing) to do that, so I deep-dove into the products that I was choosing to allow in my house and on my body, which was all I could really control. Upon hours and hours … and hours of research, I changed all of my beauty products to fragrance-free and as natural as I could find. I threw those dryer sheets and wall plugs away and found even better substitutes. I replaced all of my dishwashing liquids, laundry systems, and everything else that I could. Since I have done that, I have not had a migraine. I no longer needed daily medicine to manage my swelling, rashes, and severe migraines. They were gone.

The fact that I could control those symptoms that I was having just by limiting my exposure to these harmful irritants in our everyday lives and replacing them with better alternatives that actually are *good* for me was extremely eye-opening! That was the beginning of me realizing that using natural products actually *was* a thing, and I no longer wanted to expose my son and husband to these harmful chemicals either!

Cancer runs strong in my family lines, and I knew that if I didn't get to the root of all of this unknown dis-ease in my body, it wouldn't be good for my future health, and I couldn't teach prevention to my son. Not only did my dad struggle with cancer, but my mom and I have as well. My mom is currently fighting her second cancer diagnosis, this one deemed "incurable" by Western medicine. She is embracing the natural healing world and all it has to offer, and her mind is strong like my dad's was, so I know she will come out of this stronger than ever and with a radiant story to share. Her goal is to find natural healing that works for her specific cancer and then become a Holistic Cancer Coach to help other fighters do the same. I can't wait to see her accomplish this.

When I was 27 years old, I was diagnosed with cancer and scheduled for surgery. My mom had been using essential oils for a while and suggested I start using them right away, so I did my protocol several times a day. I was willing to give anything a shot! I was newly divorced, in a new city, and I had a young son to raise and live for. I was seeing one of the top surgeons in the nation, and when I went back in for my pre-surgery check in, he was shocked. He had never seen a tumor start shrinking on its own! The tumor had softened, and it gave better margins for a more successful surgery, and I believe that's why I didn't have to follow surgery with radiation as originally planned. I knew this gift came from God and the beautiful natural gift of essential oils that He equipped us on this Earth with.

I had to break the generational stronghold that cancer had on my family, and I knew that the way we treat our body, stress levels, and exposure to harmful things are all contributing factors to cancer in the body. So my investigation continued with even more determination.

I didn't want to be on all of these medicines I kept getting prescribed, especially if doctors didn't even know what was causing it all. I know there is a time and place for when it is necessary for some pharmaceuticals, such as immediate life-saving needs. However, in my situation, it seemed unnecessary, but it was either take the medicine, or just "keep on keeping on" the way I was. Those were the only two options that I knew at that time.

So, I went to a psychiatrist like my family and doctors had been suggesting, and she put me on two different medicines. It honestly was great at first; the first month or so I was feeling better and started to feel more in control of my life. But then the additional side effects started creeping in. The extreme brain fog was the worst for me! I'm a high-functioning, hard-working mom, and let me tell you, brain fog was NOT my friend! I kept pushing on in my holistic research, thinking, "There has to be modalities on this Earth that God created to heal us where I don't have to choose between severe anxiety and all these other symptoms or pharmaceuticals."

And so I started to slowly (at first) try the modalities I was starting to learn about.

Hot yoga was my "gateway" into the power of holistic healing. When I started realizing how my.breath (yes, just my breath alone) could control how my body responded to my thoughts, it opened a hole for me that I jumped right in. I shortly became obsessed with researching different natural modalities that weren't related to having to take pharmaceuticals, and I wanted to know all about them: the "why" behind them, the power they held, the "how" they worked, and what more was out there that I could learn about.

One by one, I said goodbye to my anxiety medicine, my depression medicine, my fibromyalgia medicine, my high-blood pressure medicine, my weight-loss medicine, and my allergy medicines, and started saying hello to hot yoga, sound therapy, energy healing, breathwork, meditation, natural supplements, whole and organic foods, life coaching, and moments of stillness.

That is now my new prescription that I have the power to control and utilize to fuel, heal, and maintain my body with. Now I am able to thrive and live my best life while sharing with others how to do the same.

As I sit here with an all-clear mind not fogged by ANY pharmaceuticals, I allow myself to release pent-up emotions that the medicines didn't allow me to have. Those emotions are natural. You should experience tears and a release when you lose a loved one or have hard challenging times in this life. That's why God created tear ducts, so that we can release the emotions boiling inside of us. But it's just that, it's releasing them. It doesn't serve our bodies any good purpose to hold them all inside and let them build. We need to use natural modalities to help us move through those emotions to come out on the other side of the release as a stronger and lighter version of ourselves.

I became obsessed with educating myself on the natural modalities available. Every available minute that I had outside of work and taking care of my family was immersed in learning and getting certification after certification along with the necessary education to become a Holistic Wellness Practitioner. The more I learned, the more I wanted to know. I became extremely passionate about receiving the education necessary to help others who may be having similar struggles along their journey. In 1 Thessalonians 5:21, it reads "*Examine everything carefully; hold fast to that which is good.*" So that is what I did, and continue to do. The more I dig, the more scripture I find that supports this holistic way of life and healing. My mission is to share these scriptures with others. That way they too can feel confident and comfortable applying these modalities to their lives.

All of these moments were important lessons in my life:

- Learning that you can't let stress continue to build or you will eventually "explode," and instead utilizing natural modalities to control daily stress.
- Utilizing the power of your mind, like my dad did, to control how your body responds to your physical and mental circumstances.
- Using natural, everyday solutions to help with allergies and antihistamines in your body to eliminate unnecessary negative effects on your physical body and mind.

These lessons all built upon one another to lead me to create my company, Be Blessed Sound Healing & Holistic Wellness, a Christ-centered and holistic approach to assist in finding peace and wellness in this busy and crazy world. We utilize the natural tools, supported by scripture, that God has blessed us with from this Earth and within our bodies. Based on each individual, we can do a combination of different options. A great starting point is with our hair tissue mineral analysis test that we use to identify and get to the root cause of many symptoms and really understand your specific body, what is impacting it, and what you can do to optimize your health. This is a shortcut so that you don't have to spend years and thousands of dollars on testing and copays to ultimately not find out what is going on in most cases like I did. Based on your results, we can then choose a combination of several supporting modalities to assist in getting your body back to the thriving state that God intended for it to be. We use multiple approaches such as Functional Medicine, supplementation, elimination, energy therapy, sound therapy, wellness coaching, herbalism, essential oils, nutrition, meditation, breathwork, and more. Our goal is to utilize techniques and therapies that will center your mind, body, and spirit so that you can find your inner peace, become a better version of yourself (for you AND your loved ones), and ultimately draw you closer to God.

I invite you to not settle for this world's "norm" of fogged brains, overly prescribed pharmaceuticals, and suppressed emotions. Instead, choose to dig into the resources available for you to feel vibrant, alive, and whole again!

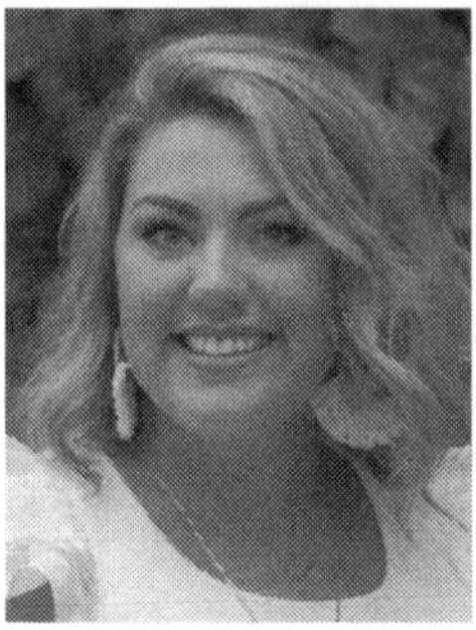

ABOUT CASEY FISK,
CSWWC

Casey Fisk is a multi-passionate Certified Alternative Healing Practitioner, Certified STORRIE Wholistic Wellness Coach™ (CSWWC) from the STORRIE Institute™, Sound & Energy Therapist, Meditation Teacher, Professional Life Coach, Vegan Nutrition Health Coach, and she has a Fully Accredited Certificate in Natural Medicine & Herbalism. As a mentor and business developer for health, beauty & wellness professionals for the past 15 years, Casey developed a deep desire for helping others, thus, her company "Be Blessed Holistic Wellness" was born. It is a Christ-centered & holistic approach to assist people in finding peace and wellness in this busy world.

She is passionate about clean toxin-free beauty and household products, clean eating, essential oils, sound healing utilizing multiple types of instruments, energy healing, holistic health, helping people as a life, business, & wellness coach and most importantly, God!

Casey is a mother and cancer survivor, being a resilient overcomer is her superpower. She struggled with mental and physical health challenges for many years until she discovered the natural methods that God created for us to utilize to heal our bodies and minds. It was life-changing, and as your Christ-centered holistic wellness coach, she shares with you natural ways to help you thrive mentally & physically and center your mind, body & spirit so you can show up as your ultimate best self for you, your family & God.

www.beblessed.today | casey@beblessed.today |
IG: @beblessed_natural_healing

UNLEASHING THE BODY'S NATURAL ABILITY TO HEAL BY ADDRESSING THE ROOT CAUSE

By: Dr. Phylicia Harris,
DNP, APRN, FNP-C, CSWWC

"Disease [is] not an entity, but a fluctuating condition of the patient's body, a battle between the substance of disease and the natural self-healing tendency of the body."
– Hippocrates

I can still vividly remember being assigned a group assignment in my nursing undergraduate community health class. Each group was assigned a low-socioeconomic community to visit to determine what, if any, health resources were readily available to them. We spent time in the community assessing their access to grocery stores with healthy, fresh food options, parks and green spaces, and even nearby health clinics and hospitals. The community lacked absolutely every resource we were looking for. It was evident in talking with individuals of the community that they lacked not only access to these resources, but also the basic understanding that their everyday choices and activities could significantly affect their overall health. They did not realize to the full extent how much their consumption of fast food and highly processed foods from the local convenience store led to disease. Neither did they realize how the simple act of taking a daily 30-minute brisk walk could benefit them in preventing disease. Our teaching on seemingly modest lifestyle modifications made such a huge impact on them, and I was left amazed at it all.

It was from this experience, which now has been more than 13 years ago, that a passion for what I called "preventative healthcare" was born. Although I was just about to begin my nursing career, I knew what I wanted most was to make a real impact and to improve the health and life of those I'd care for. For me, this had to start with preventative education. Our goal in engaging with the low-socioeconomic community was to inform them of disease processes and then educate them on the measures they could take to promote their health and prevent disease. Ultimately, our education would empower them to choose healthier behaviors and make changes to reduce their risk and severity of disease. Imagine how vital this education was for the community. While afforded little to no access to healthcare, they could be able to take control of their own health by avoiding diets lacking in essential nutrients and minerals, limiting exposures to allergens and toxins, increasing their activity levels, or just by effectively managing stress and getting adequate sleep. This understanding further confirmed the level of impact and help I wanted to provide patients. I knew it would be better achieved by addressing and preventing the root cause of disease and not by just focusing on the treatment or cure of disease. Little did I know, years later I would learn about a "root cause medicine" that resonated even more with me and my desires as a healthcare provider. My passion for "preventative healthcare" would turn into wonder for Functional Medicine and an increased desire to treat more holistically to promote overall wellness.

I learned of Functional Medicine for the first time about two years ago. My introduction to it came about while watching a masterclass of Maggie Berghoff, a nurse practitioner who successfully built and scaled an online business rooted in Functional Medicine. To this day, I honestly do not know how information about her masterclass ended up on my Facebook homepage. I had never heard of her and had not completed any research on anyone nor anything regarding Functional Medicine. Actually, the term "Functional Medicine" was completely new to me. Maggie's appearance on my homepage seemed to be random, but at the time I assumed it was probably the result of great, targeted advertising. When looking back on it, I know it was meant to be, as it was yet another experience that served to guide the path I'd journey as a healthcare provider. Maggie explained Functional Medicine as a nonconventional, science-based approach of treatment that looks at identifying and addressing the root cause of disease. She went on to explain the ways how doing so could lead to the point of reversal or possible remission of disease. The ability to truly rid patients of their ongoing and often debilitating symptoms, along with the possibility of eventually putting disease in remission, was purely mind-blowing to me, and it's what excited me most. I'd never heard anything like this in conventional medicine, where symptoms and disease are treated with medication, radiation, or surgery. Following what I was taught in conventional medicine, I'd prescribe a pill or a procedure, which downstream could lead to side effects and other dysfunction, while also only band-aiding symptoms. This is not to say there's not a place for conventional medicine; I feel it's best in acute care to quickly arrest severe complications of chronic disease and life-threatening illness. But to reverse or rid any chronic condition, it made sense to address it at its root.

As individuals, we each have unique experiences that have led us to where we are today. My story does not exactly resemble that of many others who found Functional Medicine and holistic wellness through their own personal health and healing journeys. This is true even despite the fact that I have a chronic disease. During my childhood, I suffered from asthma attacks that left me, many times, laying on the couch at my best friend's house or standing off to the side at dance practices and in gym class, struggling to get my breath. There were other times that caused a visit to the doctor or hospital. However, I did not have the knowledge at the time to seek out more holistic approaches to my asthma. What I did know was the importance of prevention. Thankfully I knew my triggers, mostly environmental irritants and intense exercise, and I did all I could to avoid them, plus I kept my rescue inhaler close by. I don't recall my doctor suggesting anything outside of this. Fortunately, my symptoms have improved to the point now that I rarely suffer from an asthma attack. However, I do wonder if there were ways I could have benefitted as a child if my doctor practiced more holistically and really dug deeper to search for the root causes of my asthma. Yes, there is a family history present. I inherited asthma from my mother, who, by the way, still suffers greatly during her experiences of acid reflux, seasonal changes, and varying temperatures in weather or her current environment. But I do not recall ever being offered any food sensitivity testing or being questioned on my eating habits or even stress and emotional health. I felt I had a great doctor, but he never educated me, or my mother, about the fact that the steroid inhaler I relied on to come to my rescue could also worsen my immunity, and in turn, increase my risk. Take a moment and imagine if these things had actually taken place. Nonetheless, this is no fault of my doctor, parents, or anyone else for that matter. My doctor practiced as he learned from the conventional standpoint; he was not trained to practice nonconventional methods as a holistic or Functional Medicine practitioner would.

And while I have a childhood history of asthma, it was more about the experiences of others that increased my interest in the practice of Functional Medicine and holistic wellness. I have seen many patients, friends, and loved ones suffer from their ongoing and progressively worsening chronic conditions. Whether it be suffering from worsening diabetes, pain from arthritis and inflammatory conditions, heart disease, or dementia, the outcome was always the same. Conventional treatments failed them as they never got to the root cause of their symptoms. As a RN, I worked over seven years in a cardiac ICU stepdown unit, with the majority of patients I cared for having presented with coronary artery disease requiring coronary stents or bypass surgeries. Again, prevention was key in my mind, and I knew there was much more we as health professionals could do before patients got to this stage of severity. How many health dollars and lost days of work could be saved if only the root cause was addressed? I have heard many stories of patients making repeated visits to the doctor with the complaint of worsening symptoms and feelings of hopelessness, just to leave feeling dismissed and unheard and with a new prescription that came with a long list of cautioned side effects. My eyes were now opened to what Functional Medicine could offer, and my patients' and loved ones' desire for relief resonated within me.

Having a heart for others, I wanted to help individuals improve their health in what I felt to be the most meaningful way. This is through educating them of the upstream, root causes of disease so that they are inspired and then empowered to take back control of their health and prevent continued dysfunction in the body. Many individuals desire to be well, but simply do not know the "how" to get well and stay well, nor the "who" to turn to that would truly listen and support. Time constrictions and other limitations often come into play when caring for patients through the conventional medicine approach. I saw this to be true in my experiences in both the outpatient and inpatient healthcare settings. In treating from a more patient-centered approach, Functional Medicine practitioners spend significantly more time with patients in order to fully listen and explore their histories and make interconnections among the genetic, environmental, and lifestyle factors influencing their health. In order to provide care in this desired manner and in a way that would fulfill me personally and professionally, I had to take action.

Ultimately, I decided to create my own telemedicine practice, Functionally Balanced Health, PLLC, where I partner with patients to determine a unique plan to help correct the root functional imbalances in their body. Inspired by a close friend and family members who suffer with chronic pain related to arthritis and inflammatory conditions, I decided to focus my services on helping individuals who deal with related debilitating symptoms. I felt the impact of their daily physical struggles when they voiced crippling pain to the point that it causes an inability to do routine activities of daily living or get a good night's rest. There is a continual, rising prevalence of autoimmune diseases. Collectively they are one of the most prevalent diseases in the United States, and the conventional treatments are costly, carry potential serious side effects, and vary in effectiveness. I aim to help busy professionals who are tired of continually suffering from progressively worsening chronic illnesses, specifically those causing debilitating pain and inflammation, find relief and an improved quality of life by addressing nutrition and gut health. Services I currently offer include support via personalized nutritional supplement recommendations, mobile IV and injectable micronutrient therapies, hair tissue mineral analysis to look at underlying nutrient imbalances, and 1:1 consultations. I see benefits in alternative treatments, and I plan to continue to adjust my service offerings based on what aligns with my patients. If what I have said and if the services I offer resonate with you, please connect with me.

My goal is to educate, inspire, and empower patients to take health into their own hands and no longer be held captive by their disease. We have the power and natural ability to heal our bodies and our lives when we address the root cause. I will leave you with a reminder and another quote from Hippocrates, which says, "Natural forces within us are the true healers of disease."

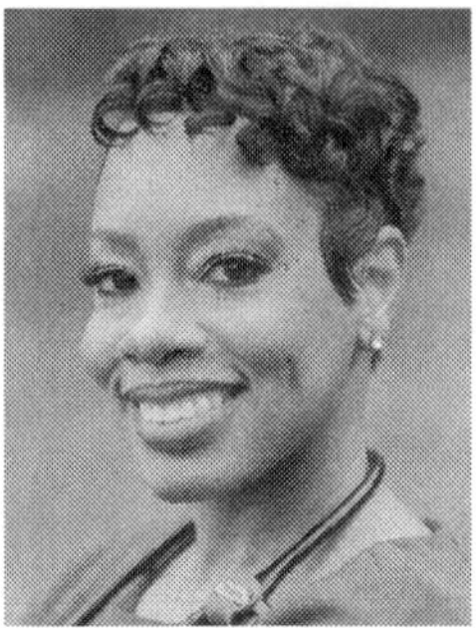

ABOUT DR. PHYLICIA HARRIS,

DNP, APRN, FNP-C, CSWWC

Dr. Phylicia Harris is a Functional Medicine Practitioner, Certified STORRIE Wholistic Wellness Coach™ (CSWWC) from STORRIE Institute™, and the founder/CEO of Functionally Balanced Health. She helps professionals suffering with inflammation uncover and correct the root functional imbalances in the body in order to improve their overall health and quality of life.

With over 12 years of healthcare experience as a registered nurse and family nurse practitioner, she's witnessed numerous patients struggle with progressively worsening chronic illness. Passionate about preventative health care and optimized health outcomes, she knew ongoing conventional treatments did not offer the best solution and decided to explore the nonconventional treatment option of functional medicine.

She has been featured in print by Authority Magazine and Memphis Voyager Magazine, and she has been a guest on STORRIE™ Podcast. Her aim is to help professionals, who are tired of continually suffering with chronic and debilitating inflammation, find lasting relief and an improved quality of life by addressing nutrition and promoting gut health using a functional medicine approach.

www.functionallybalancedhealth.com |
info@functionallybalancedhealth.com |
IG: @functionallybalancedhealth

A HEALING JOURNEY: THE FREEDOM TO CHOOSE YOUR OWN PATH

By: Britney Iannantuono,
MSN, FNP, AGACNP

"Awareness is the first step in healing or changing."
– Louise Hay

Are you a parent or professional who is suffering from anxiety, depression, and/or overwhelm? You aren't alone! Many people find themselves feeling stuck as they try to keep up with current societal demands. Learn how you can break free of patterns and beliefs that may be holding you back, and start creating a life of joy, purpose, and passion.

For most of my 20 years in the field of nursing, my passion was in acute care medicine. I knew I was literally saving lives every day taking care of patients in the ICU, but it didn't take long to realize how many people around me were suffering from anxiety and depression as they were trying to keep up with their everyday lives and the demands of their careers. I knew something had to be missing from the medical community I was familiar with since I, and many of my co-workers, had already tried traditional treatment with antidepressants and anti-anxiety medications and were still struggling. That's when I discovered Reiki. It was so different from the healing I was used to with medications and protocols. Could there be an emotional imbalance that led to physical and emotional symptoms in the body, and could realigning your energy really work? I started to really notice the benefits in my own life, and I wanted to know more!

I knew Western medicine had its place, but it was no longer enough for me. I went on to learn many other modalities to assist with my own healing process, including breathwork, frequency healing, and family constellation therapy. They were all different ways to release energetic blocks to wellness, but I found myself still struggling with fatigue, depression, and insomnia. I desperately wanted to feel better. I then discovered the use of amino acid therapy and nutrition to help with my mood disorders and cravings. I realized I could keep doing all the inner work, but if I had an imbalance of blood sugar, hormones, or neurotransmitters, I was still not going to feel well.

It takes a balance, a balance that will be different for every person based on their individual needs. We must learn to understand and process our patterns and emotions by doing the inner work. This could be through traditional psychotherapy or through other modalities like Reiki. Some will find Western medicine protocols enough, and some will seek more natural cures with diet and supplements. I knew for me personally, I needed the right balance of energy work and mindset coaching with both Western and Functional Medicine, as they all benefited me when used in the right combination. As a nurse practitioner who was ready to transition out of the stressful acute care environment, I wanted to offer clients the ability to improve their overall wellness by getting to the root cause of disease through energy work and Functional Medicine.

As far back as I can remember, I had a lot of anger. Parents and society taught us that anger wasn't allowed, that we should just hold our emotions in and move on. Don't yell, the neighbors will hear you! I learned to internalize my emotions, and when I became school-aged, I was unable to vocalize or even understand what I was feeling. I never learned how to process my emotions. I learned to hold everything in and just keep going. I became hypervigilant, to people-please and meet the needs of everyone around me in an effort to control my environment. I went on blindly living life, surviving. It wasn't until college that I realized I had no idea who I was. I couldn't make any decisions by myself, not even small ones. I was constantly worried about how my decisions would affect those around me, and I would choose based on what I thought was best for everyone else. I was stuck, frozen, lost in a swirl of over thinking or feeling numb most of the time. This was the first time I was placed on antidepressants. And it worked … for a while.

I went through nursing school, and it wasn't easy. I had to start growing up – life was getting serious. I got my first job in a neurocritical care unit, and wow, it was HARD! I had to learn to really trust myself, and that was quite the challenge for the girl who couldn't make a decision to save her own life. It took time, but I learned not only to use the knowledge I had gained, but to follow my intuition, as sometimes you just "know" when something is wrong. I stayed in that position for 10 years as I learned who I was as a person, a professional, a partner, and a mother. I met some of my best friends working there as we navigated life together. The job was hard, and life was stressful. It became the norm to be on antidepressants and to decompress with food or other substances.

It was during that time when Reiki had fallen into my life. Reiki is a healing technique in which energy flows through a practitioner's hands, activating the client's ability to heal and restore health and well-being.

For me, it became a way of life. Reiki taught me to see the world from a different perspective. By practicing Reiki on myself and incorporating the Reiki principles for mindset, intention, and presence, my life changed, my relationships changed, I changed. Anger and negativity started to be replaced with gratitude and understanding. I realized that life is a series of experiences and lessons intended to help us grow, and that emotions are messengers asking to be processed before resulting in dis-ease in the body.

As life went on, I found myself using many different modalities to manage stress as I worked through challenges both personally and professionally. I managed to get through my family nurse practitioner program, which was no easy task while working full time and being a mom. My depression, fatigue, and insomnia were worsening, but I just kept going. I had tried a few different antidepressants and sleep aids, but they would only help for a short period of time or not at all. I managed to complete a critical care fellowship for new nurse practitioners, and ultimately landed back in the same neurocritical care unit where I had grown up as a nurse. My depression and insomnia continued to worsen, and I started having terrible migraines from stress and lack of sleep, but I loved my job. My team was nothing less than amazing – they were family. I learned so much about medicine and about myself. I experienced profound shifts in self-trust, decision-making, confidence, relationship-building, and communication that affected me both personally and professionally. I was exhausted though, and I knew I couldn't go on like that much longer.

Over the years, I saw both Western and Functional Medicine providers, health coaches, and therapists to work through anxiety, depression, cravings, hormone imbalances, and adrenal fatigue. I eventually started healing underlying patterns, such as hypervigilance, overthinking, people-pleasing, and codependence. I learned these were survival techniques I likely used earlier in life, but they were now leading to worsening mood disorders and resentment and negatively affecting most of my relationships. I learned about the importance of inner child work, reparenting, setting boundaries, and developing successful relationship skills. None of this work was easy, but I knew if I didn't start to change some of these patterns, I would remain stuck.

I discovered family constellation therapy (FCT), a technique designed to identify and heal hidden personal and family dynamics that may have a negative impact on relationships and overall health and well-being. I had no idea we could carry the emotional traumas of our ancestors from up to seven generations back in our cells. The benefits of FCT were profound, releasing guilt and shame, healing relationships with people, food, substances, finances, and abundance. My perspective on life continued to shift, and I started to see my own self-worth. I learned to set and maintain healthy boundaries. I learned to speak my truth and communicate my needs more easily. I developed healthier relationships both with myself and with others. I knew I wanted to help more people who were struggling with similar issues. I started practicing Reiki professionally and incorporating what I learned during my own certification with FCT, and the testimonials were impressive. Some described sessions as an emotional reset, or a rebalancing. I was able to then help my clients develop healthier strategies to use moving forward to maintain this new state of balance. I wanted to do more of this work, but I was struggling to find the time and energy.

Things were going well, but I was growing more and more tired from the long shifts. I wasn't taking good care of my body. I needed a lot of caffeine to keep going, but I still felt tired. I would then lie awake in bed at night unable to sleep. I was stuck. It was a vicious cycle, and I didn't know how to stop it. I then discovered amino acid therapy. I started by filling out a simple mood questionnaire that I later learned was backed by 20 years of experience and was 80 percent accurate in determining depletion in blood glucose and the neurotransmitters serotonin, catecholamines, gamma-aminobutyric acid (GABA), and endorphins. According to the chart, I was low in catecholamines, which explained my lack of drive and focus and low energy level. I was low in GABA, which partially explained my insomnia, and low in endorphins, explaining why I really didn't find much pleasure in daily life at the time. I was still slightly low in serotonin, even though I was taking a prescribed medication to increase serotonin. The chart explained that craving caffeine and stimulants was likely due to low catecholamines, and that my evening cravings for sugar could be related to low serotonin. I learned how much skipping meals during my long shifts was affecting me since when blood sugar is low, the part of the brain responsible for making intelligent decisions shuts down and adrenaline spikes, causing irrational moods.

I started noticing an improvement in my mood, energy, and sleep when I started taking the appropriate amino acid supplements and getting optimal nutrition with at least 20 grams of protein every four hours to prevent dips in blood sugar. I liked that I was able to replete multiple neurotransmitters at the same time. Rapid titration was also possible since the supplements could show some improvement in symptoms within 20 minutes. This really made sense to me, and I wanted to learn more. I got certified in amino acid therapy for addiction and mood disorders through the Academy for Addiction and Mental Health Nutrition. It was the last piece I needed to complete the holistic health practice I was building. I knew it could benefit so many people by actually getting to the root cause of their symptoms.

I am a firm believer that you must take a holistic approach to heal both the body and mind. We must learn to keep our bodies in proper energetic flow so we can intentionally create the life that we desire. After years of searching, healing, and learning, I am now a Reiki Master, Certified STORRIE Breathwork Coach, and Family Constellation Facilitator. I am certified in Amino Acid Therapy for Mental Health and Addiction. I have personally used these modalities to improve depression, anxiety, insomnia, people-pleasing, and codependence. With new awareness and perspective, I am now able to live a more authentic life of joy and purpose by making decisions from a place of presence and self-trust. I recently was able to become "unstuck" and leave my busy job in the ICU to pursue my dream of helping people heal in a different way. I am the founder and CEO of Energetic Restoration, LLC, which offers a unique combination of services to help clients release what is holding them back, restore proper energetic flow, and redesign a life of joy, purpose, and passion.

Life is a series of choices. In every moment, we have the power to decide what we will say or do. By continuing to use this holistic approach to wellness, we can learn to make decisions from a place of love, or presence, rather than from our old programming, or fear. We can release the need to choose based on other people's opinions or even societal norms, for we are truly the only ones who can decide what decision or protocol is "right" for us. It takes consistent practice to quiet the mind enough to actually hear the guidance of our inner knowing. When we are truly present, we balance the overly analytical mind with our gut feeling or intuition. We can create a proper action plan, but also know when to trust and move through fear, when to ask for guidance from others, and most importantly to make decisions based on what intuitively feels most right in that moment. I knew I had reached this level of awareness when I was able to choose to leave my full-time career in the neurocritical care unit to pursue my goal of building my holistic wellness practice. I created a detailed plan to ensure success by taking a part-time nurse practitioner job with better hours and higher pay and maintaining a contingent position at the hospital while I continued to follow my intuitive guidance and create Energetic Restoration, LLC.

My journey didn't go exactly as planned, and here is what I learned. Fear will come up. You can go from feeling like you're on top of the world to feeling like you made the biggest mistake of your life. Change can be scary! But there is one thing that is worse: feeling stuck, stuck in a cycle of overthinking, or overeating, or in a job or relationship that is no longer meeting your needs. In every moment, we can decide to move toward our goals or to remain stuck in fear. Take action. Decide. Either change the situation or learn how to change your perception of it. You have no idea the freedom that may be on the other side. Be prepared to keep making decisions, as things often don't go as planned. Learn to analyze and properly prepare for anything, but always trust that your intuition will guide you in the right direction if you can stay present enough to hear it. Let new experiences in while remaining aware enough to recognize when your old programming pops up and you start second-guessing your decisions. Find what works for you to bring you back to balance, whether it is movement, music or a hobby, calling a friend, taking a deep breath, or sitting in silence. Be vulnerable, take chances, and find lessons and growth in every experience. Continue to make choices from this space, and you will create a life of exponential joy, passion, and purpose – a life of freedom.

There is no such thing as a "perfect" life. Every thought, experience, and relationship is designed to shape us into the person we are meant to be. Only when we gain awareness can we begin to understand and enjoy the journey.

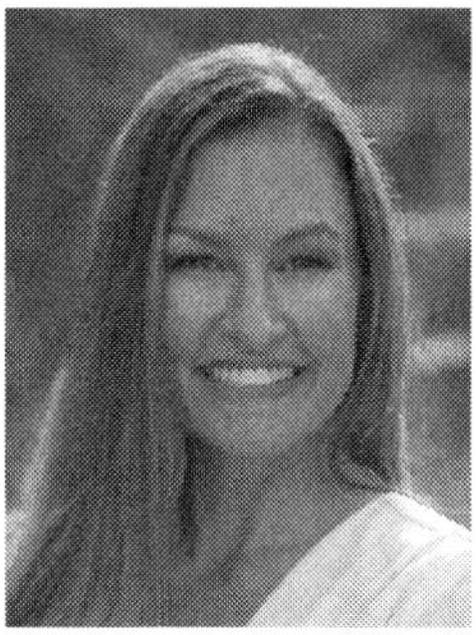

ABOUT BRITNEY IANNANTUONO,

MSN, FNP, AGACNP

Britney Iannantuono is a Certified Nurse Practitioner and CEO of Energetic Restoration. Prior to becoming a holistic wellness practitioner, Britney spent twenty years in the acute care setting as a registered nurse, then nurse practitioner certified in the areas of Family Practice and Adult Gerontology Acute Care. After her own transformation with Reiki and Functional Medicine, overcoming anxiety, depression, codependency and people-pleasing, she realized the importance of healing the person as a whole and getting to the root cause of disease. Britney left the busy acute care setting to fulfill her calling to help others release what is holding them back from living the life of their dreams by rediscovering what truly brings them joy and purpose.

Britney is a Reiki Master, Certified STORRIE Breathwork Practitioner™, and Family Constellation Facilitator. She is certified in Amino Acid Therapy for mental health and addiction. Britney is passionate about helping burned-out parents and professionals identify and release blocks to wellness, restore proper energetic flow in the body, and to make choices from a place of presence and self-trust to redesign their lives with energy work and functional medicine. Britney incorporates amino acid therapy and nutrition protocols to improve mood disorders, addiction and cravings, energy levels and insomnia by naturally repleting neurotransmitters and maintaining stable blood sugar levels. In addition to private sessions, Britney enjoys leading group Reiki and breathwork classes. Britney and her work were presented on The STORRIE™ Podcast.

www.energeticrestoration.com | energeticrestoration@gmail.com |
IG: @energetic_restoration

BREAK THROUGH TO YOUR GENIUS ZONE

By: Johnnie Kemp,
RPH

"You are greater than you think. You are more powerful than you know. You are more unlimited than you could ever dream."
– Dr. Joe Dispenza

"Break out of your comfort zone and break through to your genius zone" is not only the title of a talk that I give when I speak to organizations or at conferences, it is also key as to how I empower others to transform both their mindset as well as their physical health.

Just as my career path in pharmacy took several unknown twists and turns and provided an extraordinary level of diverse experience, my life's journey has been both wonderful and tumultuous. And I wouldn't trade it for anything.

My childhood was rather bittersweet. I grew up as an only child in a blue collar family in Mississippi. My parents loved me, especially my incredible and very protective mom. I knew she loved me, and she often gently explained that I was her "chosen child," for I had been adopted as a baby. I still fondly recall a verse from a poem my mom used to recite: "You didn't grow under my heart, but in it."

I was lucky, I often told myself. But in my heart, I didn't feel that way.

I knew I was loved, but why did I feel so unlovable? What did I do wrong? Why did my birth mother just give me away? Why didn't she want me? Why didn't she love me? "There must be something wrong with me," those voices in my head cried out. Those thoughts, those fears of abandonment and rejection, those feelings of unworthiness, gradually became beliefs that I carried into adulthood.

Fortunately, I found a refuge in science and medicine, and was awarded a scholarship to pharmacy school. Coincidentally, I poured myself into a project involving an in-depth study of the adrenal gland hormones and their effects on the body. This is something I would later reflect on as one of life's synchronicities and a preparation for what would one day become part of my purpose and passion.

During pharmacy school, I was selected for a summer internship by the National Pharmaceutical Council, and this opened doors for me to a career in pharmaceutical sales and marketing, and ultimately to becoming a clinical consultant for a company that was ranked #5 on the Fortune 500 list. I had a successful career, yet it wasn't as fulfilling as I hoped. Was I really making a difference in people's lives?

So I took a different path where I would have a more direct impact on patient care, and landed a job in home infusion pharmacy. I learned completely new skill sets like vancomycin dosing, compounding TPNs (Total Parenteral Nutrition), and programming pumps for intravenous medication administration. I really loved taking on these new challenges and stretching myself. A few short years later, I became pharmacy manager for a home infusion pharmacy for a large hospital system.

While helping my mom as she battled cancer, I became interested in assisted living facilities (ALFs). This was not my area of expertise and definitely outside of my comfort zone, but ultimately I became the owner/administrator of two small ALFs.

People sometimes ask me how all that all happened, but I didn't really find it, it found me. It was a calling, although I didn't truly comprehend it at the time. But I knew that I was truly making a difference in the lives of the elderly patients I was serving. My career and life's work now took on a deeper meaning.

My experience as a pharmacist helped with medication management and transitions of care for the residents in my ALFs. More importantly, I learned up close and personal about the challenges our frail elderly face. I've been there and shed tears with families as they said goodbye to loved ones. But I learned so much more from my residents about living, about compassion, about the power of a smile, about the gift of a hug, about being grateful for the present moment.

Although I was confident and successful in my professional life, my personal life seemed to be a roller coaster. After my first marriage ended, I found myself facing the challenges of being a single mom to three daughters. My survivor instinct kicked in, and I worked very hard to make sure I could put them all through college.

Eventually, I decided to give marriage a second try. However, after only two years of marriage, I received the shock of my life, and the tower of deceit came tumbling down. I immediately filed for divorce amid death threats, FBI watch lists, and drama that could fill an entire novel. I fled and uprooted my life, moved across the state, found a new job, and started rebuilding my life. Being a survivor just took on a whole new meaning.

Now looking back with a clearer perspective, I can see that my decision to accept that marriage proposal was influenced by what had become part of my belief system. Those voices in my head whispered that I was not really worthy of true love and real happiness … those voices that were part of a subconscious program, reminding that little girl inside of me that of course, there must be something wrong with me.

As it turned out, rebuilding my life was the best thing that happened for me. New doors opened, and walking through them changed the trajectory of my life. When we learn to overcome the stories of our past, and step into the higher version of ourselves, life is full of new possibilities.

I decided to embark on a journey of self-discovery. Along the way, I became intrigued with an expanding body of research indicating a fascinating connection between our environment, physiological responses, and cognitive functions, all tied together through the dynamic process of epigenetics. I realized that our genes are NOT our destiny. We can influence how our genes are expressing themselves so that we up-regulate the genes for health and down-regulate the genes that lead towards disease. By leveraging epigenetics, we can take control and optimize our own health.

I became a biohacker, and embraced a holistic approach to our bodies and minds as a wonderful interconnected system. This appealed to my "less is more" and "risk vs. benefit" philosophy when it comes to prescription medications. I was inspired to start a health coaching business so I could help others optimize their health and live their best lives. This has evolved into the group coaching program that I created called The Biohack Your METHOD™ where I teach women how to actually reverse biological age, while upleveling their health and their lives.

I was intrigued by research clearly showing the profound influence of meditation on our physiological state as reflected in the analyses of human tissues such as blood and saliva. Numerous studies have shown that meditation can lower levels of the stress hormone cortisol and reactive oxygen species (ROS) which are compounds that can cause damage when their levels rise too high. Moreover, meditation stimulates the release of antiinflammatory cytokines, endorphins, and neurotrophins, which are molecules that play critical roles in our immune response, pain relief, and neuronal growth.

One of the leading researchers on the effects of meditation is Dr. Joe Dispenza. His work literally transformed my life on so many levels! Dr. Joe teaches how the neurochemistry of our thoughts signals the hormones of stress to be released from our adrenal glands, and in turn, those hormones affect our gene expression. In turn, gene expression affects every cell in our bodies. Having delved into adrenal gland research for two years, I was already familiar with the science behind this process. However, the realization of epigenetics' pivotal role in our immediate well-being has truly been a revelation that holds the power to transform lives.

As hundreds of scientific studies about the effects of stress on disease demonstrate, our thoughts really can make us sick. And if our thoughts can make us sick, is it possible then, that our thoughts can make us well?

As I devoured all of Dr. Joe's books, I learned to connect with my higher self through meditation. I began to recognize those stories I had been telling myself, the ones that put up walls to protect me from being rejected, the ones that told me I was unwanted and unworthy. That was really hard! That was uncomfortable! But if I could silence those voices and cross the "river of change," I could connect with the divine energy of the universe, energy that is also inside me. Now, I have stepped into my new life as my new empowered self. I am no longer just a survivor; I am the architect of my life.

This is the journey that allowed me to discover how to break out of our comfort zones and break through to our genius zones. My goal is to empower you to embody your highest self, actually living life full-out, filled with the possibilities you only dreamed of. There is a blueprint, a formula, so that you can achieve this. It is my privilege and honor to guide you through this process to transform your life.

The core program I lead people through is called "Change Your Mind ... Create New Results," and we explore the neuroscience of change and how people can rewire their brains to create new, more productive behaviors to enrich their lives.

This program, offered only by certified NeuroChangeSolutions consultants like me, provides a unique blend of scientific theory, practical application, and personal development.

Building on the transformative power of meditation and the science of the mind-body connection, Dr. Joe developed NeuroChangeSolutions (NCS), a program designed to facilitate positive change within organizations and among business professionals. NCS offers a suite of programs aimed at fostering corporate culture transformation, improving team collaboration, enhancing communication, increasing employee engagement, and fostering creativity.

At the heart of these programs is a powerful premise: that change must start from within. Now this program has been expanded, and individuals can also take the transformative "Change Your Mind" workshop.

In my workshops, participants learn a revolutionary solution to break through to their genius zone with the Change Your Mind ... Create New Results program.

Connect with your purpose, passion, and true potential, so you can uplevel your personal and professional life.

You may feel like you are constantly putting out fires at work and at home, and you may wonder how long you can keep going before you burn out. You may be overwhelmed with juggling multiple responsibilities between work, family, and financial obligations. You may feel like you're barely hanging on.

Finally, you can get off the hamster wheel of the stressful life that is leaving you overwhelmed. You don't have to continue just living in survival mode. You just need to know *how* to remove the roadblocks that are keeping you trapped.

Imagine a work environment based on mutual respect and collaboration in a career that is fulfilling. Imagine having more time in your personal life for relaxation, joy, and even self-care.

Components that the Change Your Mind ... Create New Results program offers include:

- Replace bad habits and limiting beliefs.
- Rewire your brain for success.
- Rediscover your purpose and passion.
- Upgrade your health and well-being.
- Harness the power of your beneficial genes to elevate wellness as
- You discover how to stop living in survival mode and start living in
- creation.
- Your new life begins where your comfort zone ends!
- Discover how to tap into your genius zone!

- Become unstoppable.
- Create the life you've always dreamed of!

I'll leave you with my favorite quote from my upcoming book- *Genius Heart: Unleashing The Unstoppable You.*

"Face the uncertainty,
Embrace the unknown,
For herein lies your genius zone."
– **JOHNNIE KEMP**

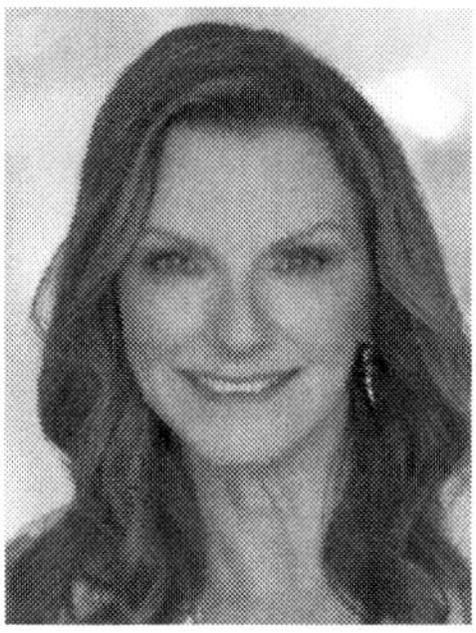

ABOUT JOHNNIE KEMP,

RPh

"Face the uncertainty, Embrace the unknown, For therein lies your Genius Zone" - Genius Heart: Unleashing The Unstoppable You.

Johnnie Kemp is a visionary pharmacist and a true catalyst for personal transformation and holistic wellness. She is also a Certified STORRIE Breathwork™ Practitioner. Her journey from a blue-collar family in Mississippi to becoming a successful clinical consultant for a Fortune 5 company, home-infusion pharmacy manager, and owner/administrator of two assisted living facilities has been marked by unexpected twists and challenges that have shaped her into the empowering figure she is today.

Throughout her journey, Johnnie has passionately explored the science of epigenetics and its profound impact on our genes. Realizing that genes do not have to determine our destiny, she became a biohacker, leveraging the power of epigenetics to optimize health and well-being. This transformative knowledge forms the foundation of her groundbreaking program, "Biohack Your Body Method," where she empowers participants to reverse biological age and achieve peak health.

Her focus on "Breaking Through To Your Genius Zone" sets her apart as a trailblazing author and speaker. Inspired by the renowned work of Dr. Joe Dispenza, Johnnie has harnessed the transformative power of the mind-body connection to facilitate positive change and personal growth.

In her "Change Your Mind... Create New Results" workshops and coaching sessions, participants learn a revolutionary approach to tap into their genius zone by rewiring their brains for success and replacing limiting beliefs with empowering thoughts. Johnnie guides them through the neuroscience of change, helping them create new, more productive behaviors and outcomes that enrich every aspect of their lives.

The "Change Your Mind... Create New Results" program offers a unique blend of scientific theory, practical application, and personal development. This transformative workshop empowers individuals to connect with their purpose, passion, and true potential, leading to profound shifts in both their personal and professional lives.

Join Johnnie Kemp on this empowering journey of self-discovery and embrace a life full of unlimited possibilities. Visit her website to learn more about her programs and discover the extraordinary potential that lies within you. Visit her website at www.mygeniuszone.com to learn more about her programs. This is your opportunity to get a free copy of her fascinating ebook, "Meditation Is The New Medication" by going to https://www.mygeniuszone.com/meditation-is-medication.

www.mygeniuszone.com | jfayek15@gmail.com | LI: @Johnnierph

TRANSFORMING THE BODY AND MIND – HEAL, RESTORE AND REVIVE

By: Dr. Stephanie Menes,
MD, CSWWC

"You cannot always control what goes on outside.
But you can always control what goes on inside."
– Wayne Dyer

Growing up in the '70s in Nigeria, I learned many things that influenced my lifestyle and career choice. The years of the '70s were mellow, relaxed, and utopian. Then children craved the outdoors, and we would run outside to play with friends and have fun, breezing through the wind like there was no tomorrow. The many games that were birthed on playing grounds were a testament to our imagination and how we employed our creative ingenuity.

Life was meaningful, and life made sense! Even as children, we were privy to the languid and relaxed ambiance of those times. The scent of the air was pure, unadulterated, and green. The wind ran through our afros, and though we were not materially wealthy, we knew that life was beautiful and there was so much more to reach out for.

These were the times we grew our vegetables in our backyard gardens, and we hardly ate processed or chemically modified food. We breathed the fresh, clean air filtered by the vegetation of the '70s. We read books to build our minds and vocabulary, and we were healthy. Yes, we thrived in good health in mind, spirit, and body.

However, the dream that was our childhood was never intended to last, and we grew up. As we turned teenagers and adolescents, we realized that the beautiful world we knew as children was changing – because the people in it were changing.

You see, this lifestyle crisis that has been given a fancy name in the corporate world – "work-life balance" – stems from the demands of an ever-changing, rapidly-paced world. Like swimming, it is easier to flow with the tide than to swim against it, so most people flow with the tide and try to conform to the ever-changing and highly unrealistic demands of a caustic world. They need to realize that these standards are ever-changing and mostly unattainable because most people believe that fulfillment and happiness come when you have attained these fluid standards. They keep trying to catch up, and their physical health, mental health, and self-esteem suffer as a result. They, in turn, burn out and become angry, bitter, and grossly unfulfilled. It is this bitterness and self-derision that affects their self-worth and, in turn, creates a conflict between their bodies and their minds. This conflict results in unhealthy lifestyle choices. It is in this space that disease thrives.

Furthermore, despite the strengths and achievements of conventional medicine, it still needs to adequately address this mind-body conflict that has paved the way for diseases to thrive in the human body. Thus

Functional Medicine to the rescue. Research shows that this mind-body conflict brings about depression – a mental disorder resulting in a loss of interest or pleasure in activities for a prolonged period. It is an illness that negatively affects how some people feel, think, and act. Also, it has been observed that people with depression or anxiety issues are predisposed to becoming obese. Obesity can result in high blood pressure, high LDL or low HDL cholesterol, type 2 diabetes, coronary heart disease, stroke, and gallbladder disease.

So while conventional medicine attacks the disease and its symptoms, Functional Medicine looks at the root cause of this disease, which could be depression, unhealthy eating habits, a sedentary lifestyle, or even anxiety, and fashions out a personalized treatment plan to modify the lifestyle habits of the patient into one that is healthier and much more sustainable.

The concept of Functional Medicine is that we can modify unhealthy habits and make them a pivotal point for healthy living. Food, for example, can be a medicine or a poison. When you eat green, organic, and healthy food, you are giving your body the much-needed nutrients it needs to thrive, but when you constantly eat junk and processed meals, food becomes a poison that makes you obese, depressed, and unhealthy. The same thing goes for a sedentary lifestyle. Sitting for long hours can cause obesity, an increase in blood pressure and blood sugar, excess body fat, especially around the waist, and unhealthy cholesterol levels, so exercise becomes a medicine for the body. This exercise boosts brain health, helps manage body weight, reduces the risk of disease, strengthens the bones and muscles, and improves overall mood.

Having practiced as a general practitioner for many years, I have come to terms with the limitations of modern medicine in healing. Also, it always amazed me that people lived longer and healthier lives before the advent of modern medicine. So, the secret to a healthy life is not necessarily the groundbreaking inventions modern medicine has achieved, but a conscious embracing of a healthy lifestyle. This knowledge has transformed my approach to my consultations with my patients. Rather than focus on an illness's symptoms, I investigate its causative factors. Is the patient depressed, obese, or a victim of a traumatic event? How have these factors affected the patient's well-being, and in what ways could they manifest as a disease? It is this orientation that I have embedded into my practice, and it has made a world of difference with my patients.

I am a firm adherent of Functional Medicine because the patient should be examined from a holistic perspective rather than addressing only the symptoms and effects of the disease. I also believe in the body's natural rejuvenating ability, which can be given a boost through healthy eating and exercise. I believe that medicine should be tailored to the very specific needs of the patient, and individualized regimens should be created to modify the patient's lifestyle. So it is this ideal that I push for as a Holistic Wellness practitioner. For me, this means preventive rather than curative medicine by adhering to a healthy lifestyle. Holistic Wellness also means using food, exercise, sleep, and healthy relationships as medicine both for the body and the mind.

"High blood pressure is a silent killer. It can strike without warning, but can be controlled with proper care and lifestyle changes."

– **Andrew Hall**

I lived a relatively good life. I grew up healthy and had an average weight with no significant health issues. My parents were healthy as well. My mum was a strong woman who gave birth to all her seven children and took great care of us. Our extended family and friends also helped us instill values we carried throughout our lives. In Africa, it is said that it takes a village to raise a child, so we grew up to value the importance of positively affirming relationships. We value the treasure that is family.

However, we observed that the silent killer of hypertension was prevalent in our family line. I observed that some uncles and aunties had this silent killer of a disease. Some did not know but discovered it later in life, while my more educated and health-conscious relatives observed the traits of this disease early on and began to manage it. One thing that I noticed, however, was that for most of my kinsmen who were susceptible to this disease, the symptoms started showing later in their lives, when they turned 60 years and above.

I didn't observe any symptoms in my health, and as a youth, I definitely was not thinking that I might be at risk for high blood pressure, so I basked in the euphoria of my youthfulness and didn't think gloomy thoughts. I met my husband, and we married and came to live in the U.S. It was here that my eating habit changed as I bought into the fast-food culture. Then I was a student and was pursuing my medical degree at the university, so my schedule was tight, and I subconsciously fell into an unhealthy eating pattern to support my fast-paced and on-the-go lifestyle. I added some weight and was highly stressed out. It was at this time that I got pregnant with my first child, and then pregnancy-induced hypertension, otherwise known as preeclampsia, set in.

Preeclampsia is a condition that causes a spike in blood pressure and protein levels in the urine. The level of blood pressure usually determines how serious the disease is. When very serious, the blood pressure can be very high, and other body organs like the liver, kidney, brain, and blood clotting system are particularly affected. Edema is a normal pregnancy symptom, usually causing swelling of the feet and ankles due to water retention; however, it could be a sign of preeclampsia, especially when there is a sudden swelling of the face, hands, and feet. If left untreated, preeclampsia can lead to severe complications such as convulsions, kidney failure, liver failure, blood clotting complications, and even death of mother and child.

Preeclampsia is particularly dangerous for the baby, because it could cause the baby to starve, thereby affecting the baby's normal development in the womb. You see, the baby in the womb is attached to an organ called the placenta. This placenta provides the baby with oxygen and nutrients from the mother's blood and removes waste like carbon dioxide by passing them back to the mother's blood. When the mother has preeclampsia, her high blood pressure can slow down the oxygen and nutrients needed to reach the baby. In severe cases, the baby can become starved of oxygen and nutrients, which usually affects the baby's healthy development. This makes it necessary for the baby to be born prematurely. Another serious complication that may arise from preeclampsia is placental abruption. This is where the placenta detaches from the wall of the uterus, and the woman experiences vaginal bleeding and abdominal pain.

I was experiencing some of these symptoms during my very first pregnancy, and I realized that as a result of not eating healthy food, a lack of exercise, and a genetic predisposition to high blood pressure, which I had ignored until it showed up in my pregnancy, I was a prime candidate for preeclampsia. The first pregnancy was not an easy one. I was overweight, had excessive fluid build-up, and was prone to headaches, dizziness, and grogginess. The doctors recommended bed rest and encouraged me to lose some weight. Eventually, I had to be induced, and I delivered my baby preterm.

This experience was a turning point in my life. I learnt the hard way the importance of watching my diet and exercising. After giving birth, I made a conscious effort to shed some weight, and I researched healthy eating habits and how to cook wholesome and nutritious meals. I began the practice of taking long walks, drinking natural fruit juices, snacking on fruits and nuts, and intermittent fasting, all of which I practice to date.

Using these methods, I have no health issues; I have monitored and managed my blood pressure levels and ensured they are within a healthy range for my age. I have also introduced these values to my husband and children, and made exercise a culture in my home. My husband also used to be overweight; now, he is within average weight for his height and has no health issues.

The secret is that these methods have aided the body's natural rejuvenation process. The body has the ability to heal by itself, but this natural ability can be impeded and disrupted when our diet is unhealthy, when stress levels are high, and when we do not exercise. The body does not need too much food. It requires natural nutrients from fruits and vegetables (this is likely why the older generations lived longer). The food we eat is mainly to aid brain function; this probably explains why the human body can function for days and even weeks without food. Also, we should consider our diet in terms of quantity and quality.

The Japanese, a people with one of the highest life expectancy rates in the world, practice a principle known as *hara hachi bu*, which proposes that you eat until you are 80 percent full. It originated in the city of Okinawa, where people use the principle to control their eating habits. Before eating, this principle advises that you look at your plate, decide how much food will make you feel full, and then estimate what 80 percent of that amount would look like – this comes to about two-thirds of the food on your plate. This principle proposes that you should stop eating when you are no longer hungry, and not eat to the point of being full and bloated with food.

Another reason this is a valid principle is that the stomach takes about 20 minutes to digest food, so if you eat 80 percent of your usual meal, you might actually be 100 percent full and not know it since your body hasn't caught up with your mind yet.

In 2019, according to research by Bloomberg, Spain was ranked one of the healthiest countries in the world. Spain surpassed countries like Italy and Japan for life expectancy. A little insight into their lifestyle will tell us why.

Firstly, they follow a Mediterranean diet comprising olive oil, nuts, fish, and legumes. A 2018 study on food and dieting closely monitored the lives of people eating a Mediterranean diet, and discovered that they had a significantly lower risk of having major diseases like a heart attack or stroke than those with a low-fat diet.

Secondly, Spaniards have a good appetite for vegetables; according to European research on Health Systems and Policies, about 39 percent of Spanish men and half of Spanish women eat vegetables every day. Also according to the health report, about 58 percent of men and 67 percent of women eat fresh fruit every day.

In addition, Spaniards are known to have close family ties. Research shows that Spain ranks No. 1 among European countries for having multigenerational homes where grandparents and grandchildren live under the same roof. Spaniards also walk a lot as the commute to work in Spain is not dependent on cars. Research shows that about 37 percent of people in Spain walk or bike to work, and only 52 percent drive.

Also, Spain boasts the highest percentage of walkers in Europe; according to research from Eurobarometer, about three out of four Spaniards reported walking for at least 10 minutes at a time, four to seven days a week – higher than any other European country. Other factors contributing to their excellent health include not living a sedentary lifestyle and making lunch rather than dinner their biggest meal of the day.

Having observed why countries like Japan and Spain rank among the healthiest nations in the world, we can confidently say that the secret is in their lifestyles and everyday habits. For them, healthy eating and exercise have become so embedded in their culture that it has been passed on from generation to generation. But how does this culture start? It starts with one person deciding to do right by their health and watching their diet while exercising. After it has proven its benefits, this habit becomes adopted by family and friends, who transmit this lifestyle to others who, in turn, reap the benefits. We have to decide to take our health seriously, and that decision starts with you.

Gina, a 30-year-old patient of mine, was grossly overweight. She is what I will describe as obese. She has struggled with weight issues all her life, and the struggle became worse when she came to the U.S. as a teenager and succumbed to the junk food culture. She ate out almost every day, hardly cooked, and ate a lot of fast food. She did not exercise, and rarely went on walks. She lived a sedentary lifestyle, had few friends, and struggled with self-esteem issues. She hardly went on dates because she never felt pretty enough, and she always lost her confidence whenever she saw trim, beautiful women. As a result, she told herself she was ugly, sank into depression, and engaged in a lot of binge eating. She got bigger, and her health and mental health suffered. Eventually, she was advised to go for surgery that would remove the fatty tissues and help her be trimmer, and she was on the verge of making this decision when a friend referred her to me for help.

When she came to me, I conducted a profile analysis and saw she had high blood pressure and weighed 250 pounds. She was grossly obese, so I started her out on medication to suppress her appetite and placed her on a 1400k calorie diet while using portion control to reduce her food intake. I recommended that she stop eating out and instead cook healthy and wholesome meals at home. I asked that she stop drinking soda (she drank two cans daily before the consultations), and recommended replacing soda with fresh fruit juices, yogurt, and water. I also recommended a lifestyle change of walking for at least 10 minutes a day, and then from there, she increased the duration of her walks until she got to an hour daily.

Prior to this time, she had joint pains and was heavily fatigued. In time and with consistency, she dropped to 194 pounds, and about six months after consultations began, she dropped to 180 pounds, bringing her closer to her weight goal of 160 pounds. Now, she sleeps better, her joint pains are gone, her blood pressure is reduced, and she feels lighter. This process has also impacted her mental health, as she feels much better about herself. She is much more confident, and has embraced the can-do spirit through the tenacity she has put into her weight loss regimen. She feels and looks more beautiful than when she first stepped into my consulting room, and now she has much more confidence in her body and curves, and her feminine pride is restored.

Rolan, another patient of mine, was morbidly obese. He had a BMI (body mass index) of over 40, was diabetic with a reading of 12.5 percent, and found it difficult to move around. I started him off with shots to control his appetite. You see, Rolan was at high risk for heart disease, stroke, and kidney damage, the doctors had diagnosed him as a candidate for borderline heart failure, and his sedentary and couch potato lifestyle was not helping in the very least. A young man in his forties, life became a burden. He constantly experienced fogginess of the brain, and his mental health and self-esteem were dealt huge blows. He lost self-confidence and had anger issues resulting from his need for self-affirmation and respect.

He was on insulin shots, and when he came to me, I stopped them and started him on Ozempic® to help him lose weight and curb his incessant need to eat. I recommended that he start with 10 minutes of walking daily, which he will increase with time, and I also gave him a thorough exposé on food and its contents. I suggested foods such as rice, beans, legumes, hotdogs, and burgers, and did a step-by-step analysis of their caloric and nutritional value. Based on this, we built a meal plan specific to him and his nutritional needs. I included fiber, proteins, and some calories while aiming to reduce the oil and fat components of his meals to the barest minimum. At some point, especially at the beginning, we had to make compromises to gradually reduce the calories while adding fiber, fruits, and vegetables. This proved challenging at first, but Rolan started this, and when he began to reap the dividends, he encouraged himself to continue until he shed a sizeable amount of weight, which brought his diabetic reading to a manageable range and made his heart healthier.

One thing I have observed is that the patient's attitude matters a great deal. Some patients try to find a quick fix for their weight issues by employing liposuction techniques, but this has side effects that include bumpy skin, withered skin tissue due to uneven fat removal, poor skin elasticity, and scarring of the tissues. The most obvious disadvantage of these techniques is that they are cosmetic and do not deal with the real issues of unhealthy and binge eating, which caused the problem in the first place. To address the real challenges, Functional Medicine asks why this person is obese. Are his eating habits healthy? Does he exercise? Is there some form of depression or self-esteem issues manifesting as obesity? After answers to these have been found, Functional Medicine now goes ahead to design a personalized treatment plan specific to the needs of the individual, readjusting this plan accordingly until the desired outcome is achieved.

So while it is a joy to work with patients who are fully cooperative and understand the gravity of their lifestyle changes, there will always be those who want to take shortcuts, and may argue with the doctor's instructions as an act of defiance. Sadly, their health gets a lot worse before they realize the implications of their decision. As a general practitioner, and with my lifestyle changes based on the ethics of Functional Medicine, I have come to realize that for us to thrive in good health, sacrifices have to be made, and we have to be intentional about maintaining good health. The starting point is usually the hardest because the body is not used to this new regimen, but we must be consistent and determined to achieve our health goals.

Also, though Functional Medicine has not been fully embraced by contemporary medicine as we know it, it has been around for a long while. It dates back to the '50s, when progressive healers started to look at alternative medicine in a new light. In that era, discoveries were made about the human body and the nutrients needed to sustain it. The University of Texas, Austin campus, under the leadership of Roger Williams, PhD and his colleagues, uncovered some secrets about the body. The B vitamins and how they contributed to boosting the human body's vitality were discovered. In time, supplement companies began to emerge to produce special supplements, and with further product development and research came potential cures and eye-opening discoveries about treating human disease based on diet and nutritional therapies. By the '80s, Functional Medicine as a profession had been launched, and this happened because a small and dedicated group of healthcare professionals started to use nutrients in the form of supplements combined with herbal treatments to proffer solutions to health challenges.

Jeffrey Bland, PhD, is accredited as the founder of Functional Medicine. He coined the term, is a leading proponent of this cause, and, to date, continues to offer inspiring lectures and is a source of inspiration to groups of natural health practitioners.

Functional Medicine falls under a group of Wholistic Wellness™ practices which comprise other healthcare practices. Some of these practices include Integrative Medicine, lifestyle medicine, Ayurvedic medicine, Chinese medicine, orthomolecular medicine, energy healing, nutrition, and herbalism.

Integrative Medicine, as its name suggests, is the practice of medicine that selectively combines some elements of orthodox and alternative medicine into comprehensive treatment plans using orthodox methods of diagnosis and treatment.

Lifestyle medicine is a branch of medicine focused on preventive diseases through self-care and positive lifestyle changes. It deals with preventing, researching, educating, and treating disorders caused by lifestyle factors. It addresses preventable causes of death, such as nutrition, physical inactivity, chronic stress, and self-destructive behaviors, including tobacco smoking and drug or alcohol abuse.

Ayurveda is an alternative medicine system rooted in the Indian culture. Ayurveda therapies, which include herbal medicines, special diets, meditation, yoga, massage, laxatives, enemas, and medical oils, have evolved for more than two millennia, and though pseudoscientific, are now embraced by the Western world today.

Traditional Chinese medicine, which has its roots in the sixteenth century, includes various forms of herbal medicine, acupuncture, cupping therapy, healing by skin scraping (*gua sha*), massage (*tui na*), bonesetter (*die da*), exercise (*qigong*), and dietary therapy. One of the basic teachings of traditional Chinese medicine is that the body's vital energy circulates through channels called meridians, which have branches connected to bodily organs and functions. This concept of vital energy is pseudoscientific. Despite this, there is increasing interest from the West in traditional Chinese medicine.

Orthomolecular medicine aims to maintain human health through nutritional supplements. This concept of orthomolecular medicine builds on the idea of the body being an optimal nutritional environment and deduces that diseases result from nutritional deficiencies in the body. Treatment, therefore, involves attempts to correct these nutritional deficiencies based on individual biochemistry through the use of vitamins, minerals, and other nutrients.

Energy healing is an aspect of alternative medicine based on the belief that vital energy flows through the human body. Energy healing aims to balancc the energy flow in the patient to reduce stress and anxiety and promote well-being. Also called energy therapy, it espouses the belief that healers can channel the healing energy into a patient to effect positive results.

Nutrition, as a tenet of holistic medicine, entails eating healthy food in its natural state for optimum health and well-being. Nutrition for holistic well-being includes eating unrefined, unprocessed, organic, and locally grown whole foods.

Herbalism is the study of botany and the use of plants for medicinal purposes. Herbal medicine, as a branch of Functional Medicine, has been used to treat and prevent diseases and enhance lifespan and quality of life.

Though the primary criticism against Functional Medicine is the lack of scientific evidence, some proponents argue that while Functional Medicine interventions like dietary supplements and lifestyle changes may not be backed by evidence, there have been studies documenting the efficiency of Functional Medicine. Another criticism against Functional Medicine is the lack of standardization, which makes it difficult to gauge the effectiveness of different Functional Medicine approaches and which may lead to inconsistent treatment outcomes. Proponents believe there will be better standardization across the board for all Functional Medicine practitioners in time and with further research.

The potential for harm resulting from unintended side effects is another area that makes conventional medicine wary of fully embracing Functional Medicine. Still, it could be argued that the same goes for orthodox medicine as a whole – that unintended side effects cannot entirely be eliminated, but can be reduced to the bare minimum.

Functional Medicine has been lauded as a medical practice that affords you more time with your doctor, drills into the minutest details of your health – thereby profiling the patient's health on an individual basis – integrates the body, mind, and spirit, and takes an interest in the patient's knowledge about themselves while proferring a non-prescription and natural approach in curing ailments.

As a Functional Medicine practitioner, I have studied and observed some strategies I have adopted into my practice that have benefited my patients. One of these is the Functional Medicine matrix, which gives a holistic view of the patient's health. First in the matrix is the assimilation process, followed by the structural integrity, then the communication, defense and repair, energy, biotransformation, and elimination – all of which cut across the patient's physical, spiritual, and mental aspects. The matrix also allows for modifiable personal lifestyle nuances such as sleep and relaxation, exercise and movement, nutrition, stress, and relationships while considering triggering events, antecedents, and mediators.

The Functional Medicine timeline takes into consideration mediators and triggers and timeline events from birth that could be responsible for the patient's well-being.

Another strategy that has proven beneficial to patients is the "GOTOIT" strategy, a simple framework practitioners employ to get to the root of each patient's dysfunction, thereby providing and applying individualized treatments to address specific cases. GOTOIT, which stands for Gather, Organize, Tell, Order, Initiate, and Track, is a teaching tool to help practitioners complete the matrix and timeline. It helps health providers establish rapport with their patients, identify unhealthy patterns, get to the root cause of their problems, and propose appropriate, personalized treatments and lifestyle modifications.

Gather: The strategy emphasizes GATHERING oneself and being mindful of the therapeutic process. It also gives priority to gathering information through questionnaires, intake forms, initial consultations and physical exams, and therapeutic relationships. The tools recommended by the Institute for Functional Medicine (IFM) to achieve this include mindful meditation, health history and intake forms, medical symptoms questionnaire timeline, chronological story, ATMs and the patient's story, ABCDs of nutrition evaluation, request and report, and nutrition physical exam forms.

Organize: This aims to purposefully ORGANIZE the salient details from the patient's narrative to see where it fits within the context of Functional Medicine. It matches the patient's presenting signs and symptoms with the details of the case history. At this stage, information is organized in the Functional Medicine matrix to show antecedents, triggers, mediators, modifiable lifestyle factors, clinical imbalances, and organizing the functional nutrition evaluation.

Tell: TELLING or retelling the story back to the patient using your own words will ensure accuracy and understanding. The retelling of the patient's story is a dialogue about the case highlights, including the antecedents, triggers, and mediators identified in the history, correlating them to the timeline and matrix. This includes acknowledging the patient's goals, identifying the predisposing factors, identifying the triggers or triggering events, and identifying the perpetuating factors (mediators). It also entails exploring the effects of lifestyle factors and identifying clinical imbalances or disruptions in the physiological aspect of the matrix. It is best practice to ask the patient to join in correlating and amplifying the story, thereby engendering a context of true partnership. Recommended tools include the patient's story reviewed and shared with the aim of integrating with the Functional Medicine perspective, personal development exercises to create and strengthen the therapeutic relationship, and reflective listening, motivational interviewing, coaching, and behavioral modifications.

Order: ORDER and prioritization come from the dialogue between the professional and patient. The patient's mental, emotional, and spiritual perspective is paramount for prioritizing the next steps.

Initiate: INITIATE further assessment and intervention based upon the above work. Perform further assessment, initiate patient education and therapeutic intervention, and refer to adjunctive care if needed. They include nutrition professionals, lifestyle educators, and healthcare providers. Suggested tools include the Functional Medicine prescription, referral for functional nutrition evaluation, ABCD order form, physical exam form, PFC-MVP biomarkers, diet, nutrition, lifestyle journal, and mindful eating.

Track: TRACK further assessments, note the effectiveness of the therapeutic approach, and identify clinical outcomes at each visit – in partnership with the patient. Recommended tools include a medical symptoms questionnaire and body composition tracking.

The Institute for Functional Medicine highly recommends the above methods and strategies, and they are being adopted by Functional Medicine practitioners worldwide.

For me, this is a calling. More than a career, I find joy in helping people live a natural and healthy life. I have seen the effects of Functional Medicine in my life, and I pledge to spread the gospel of Holistic Wellness to all who are willing to listen.

I pledge my career to helping people adopt healthy and sustainable lifestyles.

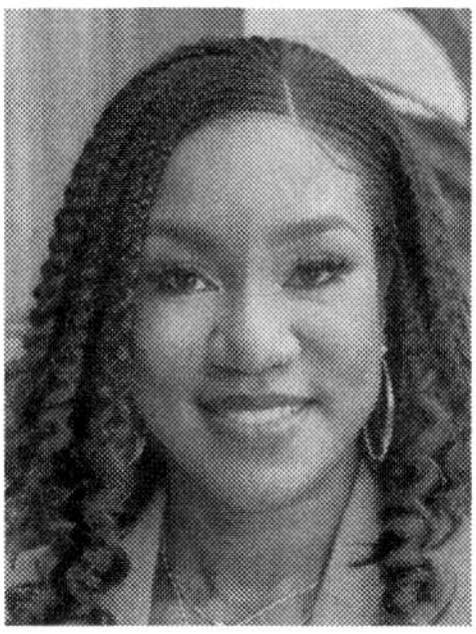

ABOUT DR. STEPHANIE MENES,

MD, CSWWC

Dr Stephanie Menes is a medical practitioner in Texas, United States of America. With twenty-two years of experience in the medical field, she has transitioned to functional medicine and wellness, having realized the power of positive lifestyle changes to ensure good health.

A graduate of Meharry Medical College in Nashville, Tennessee, Dr Menes is currently undergoing a wellness certification program at IAP College and is in the process of becoming a Certified STORRIE Wholistic Wellness Coach™ (CSWWC) from STORRIE Institute™.

Her passion for wellness was born from her health challenges resulting from being overweight and hypertensive. She was a burnt-out physician working long hours, weekends and evenings and she did not pay much attention to her physical health. She had low self-esteem due to her weight and she felt dissatisfied with herself. However, she took up the challenge of exercising regularly, eating healthy, and proactively seeking positively reaffirming relationships, and her life, mind and physique took a turn for the better. Also, Dr Stephanie Menes discovered that the conventional healthcare model restricted her ability to offer solutions to her patients the way she is passionate about without the use of medications.

The transformation she achieved from her positive lifestyle changes made her embrace the tenets of wellness and functional medicine which she reinforces with her patients, family and friends. Her consultations promote a healthy diet, exercise, meditation and positively reaffirming relationships. She believes that these can boost an individual's well-being, self-esteem and cut across the body, mind and emotions to ensure optimal health.

Dr Menes has consulted with people living highly stressful and mentally exhausting lifestyles. She seeks to address this imbalance by educating people on managing their stress levels and taking better care of their health. She is passionate about helping burnt out and busy professionals identify and embrace blocks to wellness, restore desired energetic flow in the body and mind, and guide them to make healthy choices derived from a place of presence and self trust.

She encourages her patients to be health conscious by participating in exercise regularly, practicing intermittent fasting, adopting healthy eating habits, and engaging in positively affirming relationships. She believes everyone can achieve excellent health.

Join Dr Menes as you explore your path to holistic healing, restoration of mind and body and a discovery of a revived new state of optimal and enhanced well-being.

www.healreviverestore.com | healrestorerevivewellness@gmail.com

FB: @stephanie.menes.98

TRANSFORMATIONAL HEALING: DISCOVERING HARMONY AND ALIGNMENT THROUGH LIFE'S CHALLENGES

By: Dr. Jesica Mills,
PHARMD, ND, MBA, RPh, BCES, BCLS, BCNP

"You have the power to heal your life, and you need to know that. We think so often that we are helpless, but we're not."
– Louise L. Hay

"*If I'm going to make it out of this, it's going to be because of you figuring out how to save me.*" That's the words my dad said to me after being told his recurrent non-Hodgkin's lymphoma was terminal and there were no more options. He was given less than six months to live, and I was six months pregnant with my first child, Audrey. I had just purchased the family pharmacy a few months before, and I never planned on navigating parenting and pharmacy ownership without my dad.

In 2016, dad went in for his six-month checkup with his oncologist, Dr. Morgan, who helped him "beat cancer" from his initial battle in

2011. His blood markers looked great, but Dad was having some swelling over his eye. He had gone to an ophthalmologist earlier that week, and was given some eye drops and told to not worry about it. Immediately, the oncologist sent in orders for scans, and within a few hours, he went from telling Dad he was still "cancer free" to scheduling emergent surgery to remove the tumor wrapped around the levator muscle, which is the muscle that controls lifting the eyelid.

It was no surprise when the pathology report came back and said it was B-cell non-Hodgkin's lymphoma. It was no surprise that the surgeon wasn't able to get all of it. It was surprising that when he went in 10 days later for the post-surgery follow-up, Dad reported some pain and pressure, and the doctors found the tumor had grown back and was now larger than when he originally went in. It was a surprise when they admitted him and started him on seven bags of chemotherapy that night. It was a surprise that someone who had handled a chemotherapy regimen that is known to cause severe side-effects (R-CHOP) so well during the first round of this cancer was lying on the couch and scared he wouldn't be able to take the next breath due to the side effects. It was the moment we decided that more chemotherapy was not an option, which was a hard decision to make. **Deciding to not use the only option offered, and having your life depend on it, is the moment where you find what faith and courage really mean.**

After the surgery didn't work, after the chemotherapy side effects were too severe, the only option left was radiation. Typically, this cancer type responds well to radiation, and Dad completed 18 of the 20 planned sessions. The pain, the burning, and the permanent distortion of his vision caused the doctors to stop the sessions at 18, knowing the success rates are similar to the full regimen. Dad was not going back to see if the radiation worked until after I gave birth to Audrey, so I scheduled an induction, unknowingly signing myself up for a harder and exhausting labor and delivery for my first child. **It's traumatic when you really examine the actions and risks that you will take, and the violation of your core values and boundaries to have a false sense of control and certainty in a situation**.

After Audrey was born on October 14, 2016, Dad went in and was given the news: The tumor had not shrunk, and was about the same size. There were no more options that Western medicine or Vanderbilt Oncology had. Dr. Morgan tapped Dad on his knee, with a solemn look, and gave him an expiration date: "You have less than six months, and it's time to get your affairs in order." That moment was imprinted in my dad's mind, and that day is the day that he fully accepted and received the identity of a terminal cancer patient. No matter how he would feel nor what the test results showed, any small health issue was confirmation that the cancer was growing, and his time on this Earth was limited. **With one sentence, a well-meaning doctor was able to assign him with an identity that didn't serve his healing and fractured his ability to believe his body was capable of healing.**

I remember that expectant and anxious feeling when part of your family's fate is in the hands of a medical doctor. The day we were waiting to find out if the treatment plan had worked, as well as what our future options were, I had been calming myself by taking care of my newborn. I was trying to pray and be calm and hope for the best, **having a shallow idea of what faith was, and putting my emotional regulation in the hands of a 12-day-old**. I remember getting the call, where my mom and dad wanted to tell us the results in person. I can remember every detail about that conversation in my living room, where everyone was sitting, and the clothes they wore. I now know that being able to recall everything vividly means that it was registered in my brain as a trauma, and was not properly time-stamped and filed away into the memory. It was stored in the area that puts you into fight, flight, freeze, or fawn. **It causes you to stay hyper-vigilant and constantly be looking for warning signs of anything going wrong.**

I remember hearing the news and feeling the heaviness of hopelessness in my body. I remember the confusion, the anger about how life isn't fair, and how this isn't the way it was "supposed" to be.

Grief is not something we are taught much about, especially when you are grieving the difference of what you thought life would be like, and what it turns out to be. **The suffering that we go through and self-inflict is directly proportional to the contrast between our ideal vision and our current reality.** The suffering is also optional and is what we experience only when we refuse (or don't know how) to grieve. Each human emotion can be felt and processed in 90 seconds. Any emotional response that lasts beyond that 90 seconds is the person choosing to stay in the emotional loop. We stay in these loops by attaching meaning to an outcome, chasing, forcing, judging, and projecting.

Some people would cry, grieve the situation, and then accept it, as the **liberation you seek is through the grand acceptance of where you are.** I could have felt the feelings and allowed the energy of my emotions to pass through me, but instead, I developed a skill (coping mechanism) of jumping in to fix and solve a problem for others. This is the same response that would lead to my executive dysfunction and the codependency I willingly placed myself in. I took on the challenge of beating my dad's Stage 4 terminal cancer. I researched every modality in alternative medicine, and on November 25, 2016, with my 6-week-old in my arms, enrolled in a Doctorate of Naturopathy (ND) program. I never planned on getting a second doctorate (I had earned my PharmD and MBA in 2014), but I also didn't plan on letting my dad down and allowing cancer to win without showing up to the fight. **The most intense challenges in my life have usually come from something not seen and not planned for**, which makes you hesitant to live in the present moment (the only moment you have power, since it's the only one that is within your control).

As I would learn, we would implement. I started learning the foundations of health, including sleep, breathing, drinking enough water, pH balancing, and eating to fuel your body. I learned about the amazing survival mechanisms of the human body, and the innate intelligence our Creator gave our body. **It turns out, having high cholesterol is not due to a statin drug deficiency,** but instead is a symptom of a biochemical process that is not functioning correctly, an organ or two needing support, and some lifestyle changes that need to happen. This was a foundational shift in my perception of what role in healthcare I wanted to participate in. My dad had been a pharmacist for over 55 years, and was always interested in natural and alternative medicine, so we were both learning and unlearning some key truths together about what health really was.

He was willing and eager to implement most changes, including changes to his diet, supplements, and changes in his habits, but the hardest piece was the mindset. People do not understand the true power of our words, and the impact they have on people, especially when we wear a white coat. The expiration date of six months from the oncologist was an anchor that was just too heavy to allow for the belief in true healing. **"There is no medicine like hope, no incentive so great, and no tonic so powerful as the expectation of something tomorrow." Orison Marden**

From following foundational health principles, plus using targeted nutrition and supplements, my dad had more energy, felt better, and made the declaration a few times that he no longer had cancer. He lived past his expiration date of six months, and then a year later, went in for a PET scan and was declared cancer-free. He saw his second granddaughter born in November of 2017, and was grateful for every day he had, as by all accounts he was living on bonus time.

In the spring of 2019, walking to the mailbox, Dad had a tick land on his arm and seize there. The tick was not discovered for 24 hours. Dad removed it, and took the one dose of antibiotics prescribed for one day. A few months later, he started to have strange bumps appear on his legs. They didn't itch, but they would grow larger, and didn't go away. He decided to go to Vanderbilt and see a dermatopathologist to determine what it was. The pathology report said "PCDLBCL-LT?" and I remember thinking I had never seen a question mark in the diagnosis line of a pathology report before. The seven dermatopathologists at Vanderbilt had not seen it before, and we found ourselves facing an "exceedingly rare and very aggressive" terminal cancer for the third time. **What you don't find and treat at the root level can always come back.** Dad had the lifetime limit of rituximab from his first round of chemo in 2011, so we found ourselves needing to create a plan without any guidance or options from the medical system. Dad had become lax in his lifestyle, as we typically will revert back to our comfort when we think it is safe to do so. **The process of healing has to be integrated into your identity and your health will always be reflective of your habits. If it isn't sustainable, it won't be successful.**

We started to get back on a strict regimen, and using the supplements that worked the first time in 2016. What I didn't know about was the impact that heavy metals in your mouth and root canals had on the body. I didn't recognize the importance of having a healthy gut to allow the immune system to function. I didn't consider my dad's decades of being a farmer who used glyphosate pesticides on his thousands of acres. I didn't know about stealth pathogens, Lyme disease, chronic EBV infections, and how to fully support the immune system when it was so overwhelmed it could no longer function. I remember having a conversation with my Creator in my basement, after talking to Dad and seeing his wounds from the tumors that kept growing larger on his legs. The feelings of futility, hopelessness, not being enough, not doing enough, and the anger of why good people are suffering in this world caused me to ask/shout, "Why isn't anything working this time?!?" In a moment of heavy stillness, I heard, "There was a tick bite this time."

I immediately searched if this type of cancer was associated with Lyme disease. There were seven studies (all in Europe) that showed a link to B. burgdorferi. I knew nothing about Lyme disease, except the day in pharmacy school that we covered it. I thought it was eradicated with an antibiotic. I had heard of some of the stealth pathogens, like Bartonella (cat scratch fever and trench fever), but never knew mycoplasma could be a co-infection. I had never heard of babesia, anaplasma, or ehrlichia. I didn't know that standard blood labs have a false negative rate of up to 50 percent due to the disease itself inhibiting the immune system. I didn't know that the existence of chronic late-stage Lyme disease (which we learned about in school) was controversial and not widely accepted. I didn't know there was another set of guidelines from the International Lyme and Associated Diseases Society (ILADs), that does make recommendations from actual evidence, and I didn't know the true prevalence of it. I decided to start learning; **I felt as if it was all on me** to find the solution to save my dad.

We opened a Functional Medicine family practice in October of 2019, and I started traveling to be in the rooms where people who had beat cancer and Lyme disease were. I went to California to a conference called The Truth About Cancer, finished my in-person testing for my

ND in Texas, flew to Boston to attend the ILADs practitioner training and become a Lyme Literate Practitioner, and flew back to California to teach pharmacists about CBD and the endocannabinoid system, all in eight weeks, while our medical practice was opening and seeing patients. **The rarity, the aggression, the fact that the enemy (cancer) was visible and external this time, it all led to a frantic search for answers, which caused the abandoning of the foundational truths for a healthy lifestyle.** When you are exhausted, overexerting yourself, overidentifying with being the problem-solver, and/or overly attached to an outcome, you lose your foundation as well. You don't make smart decisions, and your judgment becomes questionable. You jump from one thing to the next, you become impatient, you miss out on being in the present moment, and even the moments you want to feel joy, you can't, because you are living life trying to be 10 steps ahead. The present moment no longer feels safe. You go from the person who stares Stage 4 cancer in the face to the person who cannot get out of bed.

Being the person who can't get out of bed causes an issue when you have been working full-time as a pharmacist, being a mom of two kids under 2 years old, owning a pharmacy and medical practice, and seeing patients as a Naturopath, while trying to stay married, helping your husband through nursing school, being the sole provider for the family, finishing your second doctorate, speaking at professional conferences, attending Masterminds and showing up as a mentor and consultant for clients, and attempting to defeat terminal cancer for the third time. I call this season "trying to be everything for everyone." **When you try to be everything for everyone, you abandon yourself and forget you have needs.** I was able to help over 200 patients during this time. I helped my patients reverse autoimmune diseases, become and stay pregnant and birth the babies they had wanted for decades, come off the medications they no longer wanted to take, heal relationships between teens with mental health challenges and their parents, order the labs that found the cause of their symptoms, and be the provider who listened and gave them the root causes of their issues, including the validation and acceptance that they weren't broken. **I was able to provide hope to those who had lost it, even when I was losing hope myself.**

I remember the day I was talking to my healer and coach (Chloe Lozano) after my travels. I was trying to find the solution to a minor problem with staff at the pharmacy, and was really focusing on it. She asked me, "What is it that you are avoiding because you feel you can't control it, that is causing you to want to control the actions of those in your life?" I said, "I'm scared that my dad is really dying this time, and I can't save him." It was an automatic response that came out of my mouth without me even meaning to say it, and then the emotion of that fear washed over every cell in my body. I cried. I grieved. I didn't stop feeling that feeling for 24 hours. It was like every instance of feeling that fear since 2016 caught up with me, and my body was finally able to process it and let it out.

We had our family Christmas, and Dad's health kept declining. I had reached a point of acceptance that we had all done the best we could, and that Dad was tired. We were all tired. I found out that I was pregnant unexpectedly at a business conference in March of 2020, and I remember Dad's laughter when I called home and told my parents. He told me this time it would be a boy. Dad passed away at home, exactly how he wanted to on March 9, 2020, right before the world went through COVID. I didn't understand it at the time, but now it was a great lesson in timing. I can't imagine the trauma of him needing medical care during the time of COVID, seeing the world politicize a virus, and I'm so grateful we were able to be one of the last three public funerals before those shut down.

I'm grateful that he was able to know about his third grandchild (John, indeed a boy), but never had to know what COVID was.

Being pregnant and grieving my dad while the rest of the world changed due to a virus, and making the changes needed for our staff at our businesses, was enough to make me lose any remaining foundation I had after years of trying to beat terminal cancer. Grief is not linear, just like healing isn't. You have some days that you are drowning in your emotions and pain. I had to find a way to process it, as my typical coping mechanisms were off the table. I couldn't travel because no one could fly, I couldn't use alcohol or any substances to numb the feelings (I was pregnant), and I didn't have the energy to overwork. **I had to rewire my thoughts, allow emotions to flow through me, and I had to find gratitude and the courage to see life differently.** I realized the number of patients I helped due to the knowledge I learned, the mentors and connections I made, the amazing vacations and memories we had with Dad for four years instead of six months, and how intentional every moment I spent with my family was.

When you have faced your biggest fear (being abandoned and losing a parent), you have built up a resilience and a strength that allows you to face uncertainty and fear in a different way than most people can. You don't get shaken as easily, and you show up to the challenges differently. **You make the choices that are in alignment with who you are.** You decide to have a homebirth in 2020, and realize you were capable all along. You decide to offer rapid COVID testing when no one else is willing to in your community. You agree to see patients in person who need you. You research and learn all you can about a novel virus, and find ways to decrease furin, to block the TMPRSS22 and ACE2 receptor binding, and create a recommendation set that keeps the 3,800 sick patients you saw out of hospitals, not on ventilators, and all alive. **You learn how to**

face challenges and create solutions. Then one day, there isn't a dying parent or a novel virus, and **you realize that you've been so busy saving everyone else, you now need to save yourself.**

The whole time I was running around searching for a cure for cancer, then Lyme disease, then COVID, I was losing pieces of my foundation and overgiving. I would rush to save, abandon my needs, not receive the gratitude I thought I was owed, become upset, and give all of my power away. It's called codependency, and a trauma triangle that cycles until you stop it. I forgot how to ask for what I needed. I falsely accepted that I was sometimes too much for people, while also not enough. I became a perfectionist. I craved validation and affirmation, and sought out heightened feelings and experiences to make me feel alive. My body was used to running from crisis to crisis, and the chemical cocktail our adrenals make in that state. I was people-pleasing as a way to validate my self-worth. I got three board certifications in one month, so I now have 26 letters after my name (which is visual proof of my hyper-achieving coping mechanisms). I would take everything personally, such as an employee putting in their notice, and would create stories that centered around my limiting beliefs, using others' actions as evidence of its truth.

Since November of 2022, I have been in a transformational growth period, where I am discovering the different facets of myself such as my inner child, my nurturing adult, and my sacred rebel, and learning how to heal and integrate these parts of me. I was never not enough, my actions just weren't always appreciated. I was never unworthy, I just wasn't asking for what I needed. I've gone to a healing medicine retreat in Costa Rica, took a transformational leadership course where I learned the principles of Shamanism, have done Neuro-Linguistic Programming (NLP) and timeline therapy, and learned how to respond from my sage perspective instead of being hijacked by any of my self-saboteurs. I've fully committed to start co-creating this life, instead of just responding to it, to find neutrality, and to leave behind the limiting beliefs and the pain, while carrying forward with wisdom. A mentor told me, "**At the end of the day, all of this healing, it really comes down to learning how to love yourself, and give yourself radical self-acceptance.**"

When leaving behind so many limiting beliefs, I found the medicine I needed, which was to go back to creating the foundation. **If you don't get to the root, the issues will just keep coming back, even if they appear slightly different.** I had to make the decision to heal my inner child, to truly embody what I help my clients do, which is to meet my body's physical needs: prioritizing sleep, eating nourishing foods, drinking enough water, getting enough physical movement to allow my life force energy to flow through and feel strong and capable. **I had to learn how to set internal and external boundaries.** I went back to the *Four Agreements* by Don Miguel Ruiz for my communication, and created the habits that serve me like deep breathing, not overconsuming, dry brushing, intermittent fasting, and creating the time and space for me to check in with my body and myself every day. I had to enforce those boundaries so that my inner child knew they could trust my nurturing adult self, and choose to respond in functional ways rather than impulsively. **I had to make every choice and commit every action with intentionality** – such as, "What am I taking in?" and "What am I releasing with each breath?" **I had to create the safety within myself, and learn how to provide myself with what I needed.**

I'm so grateful for the lessons and experiences I have had, as they have provided me with so much wisdom and tools to empower my patients with. Since I started seeing patients in 2017 at Owensboro Family Pharmacy and Wellness, I have held over 7,500 appointments, and have witnessed some miraculous healing. I have seen the reversal of chronic conditions from diabetes to MS to psoriatic arthritis, given terminal cancer patients years of life past their "due date," helped over 20 women who were told they were infertile conceive and birth babies, ordered the labs for thousands of patients who showed their antibodies to their thyroid, chronic EBV, and Lyme disease testing, and recommended foundational lifestyle changes with short-term supplement recommendations to address the root issues. I've helped dozens discover the mold, radon, and VOCs in their homes, balanced hormones, helped couples communicate and reconnect by addressing their physical intimacy issues, increased their energy, improved their sleep, helped their kids focus, and supported the parents in making empowered decisions they felt were best for their kids. I've helped save gallbladders, detoxed livers and heavy metals, helped clients regain cognitive function and relieve brain fog, and have helped people walk through the darkest times in their lives as a guide and facilitator for change.

The real secret of how I assist in transformational healing is to be able to provide hope. I empower your decision to change your habits by showing you that you have the power to co-create the life you desire, fully educating you on your options, teaching you how to listen to your intuition, fostering trust with complete honesty and authenticity, holding space for your healing, meeting and fully accepting you where you are, and congratulating you on having the courage to begin the journey of healing.

You might come in an attempt to try and lose weight, balance your hormones, get better sleep, feel less pain, or just because you don't want to take all of those medicines. Beneath that, there's usually a disempowering experience where you didn't feel heard or understood by a previous provider you went to, and hopelessness set in. But **something is telling you that life doesn't have to be this way. Your highest self knows the**

suffering is optional, and you have been wanting someone to show you that healing is possible. It is possible, your symptoms are your body communicating to you that it's time to do something different, for **you have grown as we are supposed to**, and your habits and choices and thoughts are no longer serving you. **You aren't broken, you are experiencing the one constant thing in this life, which is change**. You can choose to see your current challenges as an opportunity to **come into alignment and harmony with who you really are.**

"Be confused, it's where you begin to learn new things. Be broken, it's where you begin to heal. Be frustrated, it's where you start to make more authentic decisions. Be sad, because if we are brave enough we can hear our heart's wisdom through it. Be whatever you are right now. No more hiding. You are worthy, always." – S.C. Lourie

When you feel that the suffering is too great, and that something has to change, I'll be here, ready and willing to inspire, encourage, educate, and empower you. **You are always worthy, and the only moment with any power is the present moment. You could do something in every instant that can radically change your life.**

"Happiness turned to me and said – 'It is time. It is time to forgive yourself for all of the things you did not become. It is time to exonerate yourself for all of the people you couldn't save, for all of the fragile hearts you fumbled with in the dark of your confusion. It is time, child, to accept that you do not have to be who you were a year ago, that you do not have to want the same things. Above all else, it is time to believe, with reckless abandon, that you are worthy of me, for I have been waiting for years.'"

– Bianca Sparacino

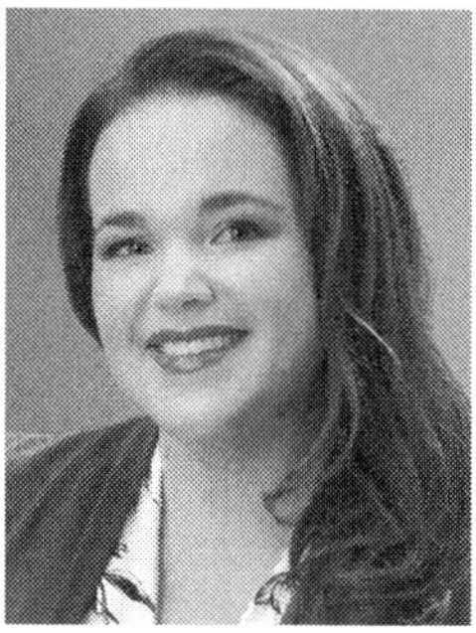

ABOUT DR. JESICA MILLS,

PHARMD, ND, MBA, BCES, BCLS, BCNP

Dr. Jesica Mills is a Pharmacist, Naturopath, Healer, Educator, Speaker, Functional Medicine Practitioner, and Pharmacy Owner, with a mission to educate and empower everyone she meets on the journey of wellness.

Dr. Jesica received her Doctorate of Pharmacy and MBA from Sullivan University College of Pharmacy. After graduation, she returned to her home town in Owensboro, KY to practice pharmacy with her parents, Don and Daisy Thomason. In 2016, Dr. Jesica purchased the pharmacy and began Owensboro Family Pharmacy. Jesica continued her parent's tradition of providing every patient with customized and compassionate care, while offering expanded services and products. Jesica finished her coursework for a Doctorate in Naturopathy, and sees clients for wellness consultations, genetic testing, weight loss, infertility, lab interpretation, and wellness regimen planning. Dr. Jesica and Owensboro Family Pharmacy have won many awards and distinctions including the Kentucky Pharmacist Associations Distinguished Young Pharmacist of the Year 2018, Reader's Choice Gold Pharmacy 2018 and 2019, Spirit of

Kindness Award, Chamber of Commerce's Emerging Business of the Year 2019, and National Woman Pharmacist of the Year 2019. In 2019 Jesica opened a medical primary care practice with her husband.

She is passionate about helping independent pharmacies thrive and adapt to new challenges, growing her businesses to educate and empower her patients, and spending time with her husband and three children.

https://bookwithdrjesica.as.me/schedule.php | jesica.1120@gmail.com | FB/IG/LI: @jesicamills

FINDING MY PURPOSE WHILE CHASING THE STATUS QUO

By: Dr. Anna Nguyen,
PHARMD, MBA, CSWWC

"Your life does not get better by chance, it gets better by change."
– Jim Rohn

The traditional healthcare approach often focuses on treating symptoms rather than addressing the underlying root causes of the health issue. Thus far, this is what I was trained to do as a pharmacist for 17 years. I graduated from pharmacy school in 2006, and have only worked as a retail pharmacist since then. Sometimes when I attended my mom's physicians' visits, I questioned their treatment of care, yet I couldn't blame them. The healthcare system has failed to mentor physicians about the beauty of alternative medicine and its positive effect on better patient outcomes rather than just managing the symptoms. Instead, the system is so broken that conventional practitioners rely on third parties to treat patients in order for the insurance to reimburse them. My mom had a long list of medications that her doctor would always keep adding to. It was a scary thing to see since the list of 10-plus medications took up an entire

8x10 sheet of paper. With the healthcare industry being a trillion-dollar company, it has failed to treat us as whole, but instead has trained clinicians to treat the disease by prescribing more pills, thinking it will solve the problem. I have realized that I am part of this system that doesn't do justice to educating others how holistic interventions are powerful tools that can heal the body.

I was very fortunate enough to have parents who truly cared for my siblings and me by focusing on our well-being and education. My parents worked hard for their money, and always valued every dollar as they lost everything when they immigrated from Vietnam to Canada. I never knew much about my parent's upbringing, as they protected my siblings and me from their horrific experience when the country was taken over by communists. When they opened their first business in the United States, they made sure we wouldn't experience the same struggles they did, and provided everything we needed so we could go to school, get a degree, and have a good job. I am sure the long hours of working as business owners and adopting the American lifestyle affected their health and the way they lived their lives in some way. But never did I hear my parents complain as they continued to work hard and support us the best they possibly could. My siblings and I were so young and unaware that my parents just wanted to raise us to have a better childhood.

The moment I got accepted to pharmacy school, it was a proud day for my parents. As a 22-year-old, life was good. I moved to St. Louis in Missouri, attended pharmacy school, and lived like any pharmacy student: happy, carefree, meeting other students from different states, and getting through all the bookwork. Two years later, a very unexpected thing happened that would change my outlook on life. My dad passed away from a hemorrhagic stroke at the age of 58. My family was in shock. Although I knew he lived with type 1 diabetes for years, he eventually developed kidney failure. We were told that his health would get better once he started dialysis and that he could start adding protein into his diet. In our minds, we thought the healthcare system was truly looking out for my dad and things were going to be as normal as possible, or at least that's what I wanted to believe. At the time, I thought that his diabetes was primarily genetic, and that eventually, like we were taught in school, complications would generally develop. Once those complications developed, as clinicians we needed to find ways to control it by giving medications. When I graduated from pharmacy school, I told myself I would help others who were in a similar situation, and hoped with my pharmacy background it would help save more lives and help patients live a better life.

Seventeen years later, I am still working as a retail pharmacist. Pharmacy as an industry just isn't the same as it was back then. It is getting more stressful and more competitive to fulfill what corporate America wants, which is to maximize profits on selling drugs that eventually become ineffective for the long run. I saw patients as just a number. Retail pharmacists are not given enough help, but are also serving as a sales cashier and a technician, in addition to their work as a pharmacist. I didn't want to see it that way, but being a pharmacist in this lifetime got more complicated in that counseling patients on their medications focused on drug name, directions, and the basic side effects, and nothing more. It was more about chasing the metrics and less about patient care. More work was being added to our plates, and it became so unfulfilling and redundant working as a pharmacist that I almost wanted to quit. But I knew I couldn't, because I asked myself, "What else am I going to do instead?" All too often, I would see patients picking up boxes of insulin along with more medications added to their list while their shopping carts were full of junk food. I thought to myself, "This is such a bad vicious cycle that keeps getting worse."

I continue to work as a retail pharmacist, but what eventually triggered my brain to think outside the box is when my mom had an emergency gallbladder removal. Upon the discovery of a failed gallbladder, she had to get a stent placed soon after her procedure. Even though it seems to be the norm to have both procedures done in this current healthcare industry, I knew it still wasn't right. Prior to this emergency admission, she experienced pain in her chest, vomiting, and pain on her right side. Initially, I thought she was just experiencing acid reflux, and so did her doctor, who ended up prescribing heartburn medications. But her hospital stay revealed more issues. Those chest pain symptoms and vomiting were a possible precursor of a heart attack. Luckily, the doctors were able to catch it before it worsened. It was during the pandemic when she entered the hospital. During that period, the hospital only allowed visitors to stay for a certain number of hours. I went to visit my mom every single day until she was discharged, but during my visit, I discovered a heart-wrenching picture of life in the hospital. I would see patients laying on the hospital bed getting blood drawn every hour, eating hospital food while watching TV alone, or just looking lonely and miserable. It was a dark moment, because I would picture my mom lying in bed by herself with no family around and a constant stream of nurses or doctors going on their rounds, discussing with each other what medications my mom should be on and whether they were appropriate. It made me realize that the healthcare culture needs to do better. Too many patients are entering the hospital for similar reasons, and time and time again, the current system only concentrates on treating the symptoms. This is just a BAND-AID®, folks! Although I believe the current system is appropriate for treating acute issues, I don't believe it will help the outcome for long-term care.

After the health scare with my mom, I knew I had to make a change and further investigate my mom's health issues. I had to be her "doctor."

Along with my own health struggles, I investigated holistic interventions and researched what I thought could help prevent or address any disease state. I became more intrigued with the information as I discovered well-known clinicians and their views regarding Functional Medicine. I'd listen to their podcasts, read their books, or follow their social media. I wanted to know more, and when they say "knowledge is power," it is truly right. It was a proud moment when I knew I wanted to be a Functional Medicine practitioner. If years ago I had known more about the power of Functional Medicine and how well the body can heal itself, maybe my dad would still be around, and my mom would not have had to endure the painful discovery during her hospital stay.

As I journey through this new chapter in my career, I have an appreciation that self-care is vital to care for another one's life. The cliché of "health is wealth" may seem overrated, but it is a phrase that truly resonates with me. I hope as I go on into this new path, my goal is educating and spreading the word on how the body can truly heal itself if we put our minds to it. What I know now is that the quality of a person's life is infinitely more significant than simply the number of years one lives. That to me is Functional Medicine, which is my primary focus to address health issues rather than relying on the traditional medicine that seems to have failed majority of Americans.

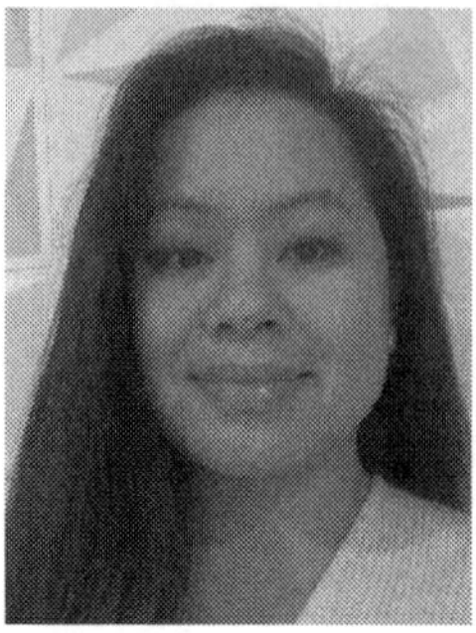

ABOUT DR. ANNA NGUYEN,

PHARMD, MBA, CSWWC

Dr. Anna Nguyen is in the process of becoming a Certified STORRIE Wholistic Wellness Coach™ (CSWWC) from STORRIE Institute™. Over the past decade, Anna received her Pharm D. degree at the St. Louis College of Pharmacy, a certificate from the Institute for Integrative Nutrition, and decided to get her MBA at the University of Nevada, Las Vegas during the COVID pandemic. She is passionate about helping others, wanting to live a healthier lifestyle and to apply alternative medicine that predominantly achieves results. She has seen how conventional medicine has negatively impacted her own family member's health as well as her own. Most importantly, she strives to educate others about the wonders of Functional Medicine and the amazing results she has followed from other holistic clinicians.

Dr. Anna has worked in the pharmacy retail setting for about 17 years and knew "popping a pill" everyday wasn't the answer to the problem. She believes that knowledge is power and learning is a daily task that should be practiced until the very end. She is excited to start this new chapter in her career and hopes that her learning experiences will open up more discussions on how thinking outside the perimeter will help us grow for the better.

annalinh526@gmail.com | IG: @dr.annalinh

WELLNESS IS NOT GIVEN, IT IS EARNED

By: Dr. Alaina Olenik,
PHARMD, BCACP, CDCES, CPP, RCPC, A-CFHC, CSWWC

"Wellness seeks more than the absence of illness; it searches for new levels of excellence. Beyond any disease-free neutral point, wellness dedicates its efforts to our total well-being – in body, mind, and spirit."

– Greg Anderson

In 2014, I was just starting a new fully clinical ambulatory care pharmacy position, having transitioned from a practice faculty position at a school of pharmacy. While I was excited, I was finding myself to be fatigued far too often and having sporadic feet and leg cramps. When they did occur, they were so bad that they would get me out of bed at night crying in agony. Filling the bathtub with several inches of hot water and standing in it was all I could do to get the cramping to stop. I went to my doctor, who ordered all the lab work I asked for, including some Functional Medicine labs. I was warned I might be charged for them as my insurance may deem them unnecessary for the diagnosis code being billed for the visit. My doctor told me to start taking prescription high-dose vitamin D and oral OTC B12 for my fatigue. I took one OTC dose of 5,000 IU of vitamin D, not even the 50,000 IU I had been prescribed, and thought I might die. I got the most intense feet and leg cramps I have ever experienced in my life that night. I was crying, hyperventilating, and writhing on the floor in pain, barely able to make it to the bathroom to turn on the hot water for my usual remedy. I could not sleep after the incident, fearing the cramps would come back.

As I lay in bed, I began researching why this was happening to me. I discovered I was likely deficient in magnesium. It turns out that your body requires magnesium for multiple steps of vitamin D metabolism. Even though my serum level of magnesium was normal on the labs my doctor had ordered, my intracellular levels were clearly lacking, and taking the vitamin D worsened my magnesium imbalance. I started taking magnesium malate, and within days I felt like a new person. It was like some switch had just been flipped, and I started to feel so much better. Intrigued that something so simple could make such a big difference, my eagerness to learn more snowballed.

I sought out a hair tissue mineral analysis (HTMA) specialist to find out if heavy metal toxicity might also be contributing to my fatigue symptoms and to see what else might be out of balance. Among some of my imbalances, my aluminum and bismuth levels were abnormally high, which led me to completely overhaul my beauty and self-care products. I immediately stopped using the majority of my current products and sought out clean-beauty brands to replace all my old favorites. I stopped drinking or eating anything out of aluminum cans. In struggling to find other sources of aluminum I might be inadvertently exposing myself to, my tea was the only other logical dietary source I could identify. I don't drink coffee. I am a tea drinker, and I mean multiple cups of brewed plain hot tea daily. I replaced all my favorite teas with higher quality organic alternatives to replace the lower quality teas I was consuming that were more likely to be grown in soil contaminated with heavy metals.

I admittedly am not someone who loves to exercise in the conventional sense. I played sports in my younger days, but always hated running. My exercise had dwindled to virtually nonexistent as my energy levels declined. I couldn't remember the last time I really broke a sweat, and I learned about how detrimental this could be for the body. Our skin, after all, is our largest elimination organ. I started learning about various biohacks, and became extremely interested in infrared sauna therapy and the health benefits it offers, including heavy metal detox. I invested in a portable tent-style infrared sauna. As I began using my sauna, it took me at least five sessions to actually break a sweat. I was shocked that I was not able to tolerate the sauna for more than about 10 minutes when I first started using it. More than six years later, a typical sauna session for me now is 20 to 30 minutes, and I start sweating within a couple of minutes. All healing takes time, and I can certainly attest to that.

On my path, I stumbled upon the Root Cause Protocol, and found myself enamored with it and the research behind it. I started to follow it, and saw so much improvement in my own energy levels I decided to go through the Root Cause Protocol Institute training to have an even better understanding of why what I was doing was helping so much and to be able to offer assistance to others. I also discovered EFT (emotional freedom technique), also known as tapping, to be essential. Being able to free myself from negative emotions that I didn't even realize I was still holding onto, that were affecting my mineral balancing, has made a huge difference in my overall wellness.

From elementary school all the way through high school, I was bright, and school came easy to me. I was interested in math and science more so than any other subjects, and enjoyed helping others and wanted to make a difference. Healthcare at the time seemed like a logical choice to pursue, but I was a little squeamish, and didn't love the idea of being a physician or a nurse for that reason. I ended up believing pharmacy would be a great fit for me. I made it through school and graduated with honors before moving on to residency. I did an ambulatory care-focused residency, and spent my days working with patients with chronic conditions. While I learned a great deal and was grateful for the experience, it always bothered me that so much of what we did was discernibly segmented. We were exceedingly focused on the medications the patient was taking and what needed to be adjusted or added to get their problem under control. We never really took the time to focus much on the lifestyle aspects other than to give limits on how much salt they should consume a day or how much to restrict their carb intake. Even in a multidisciplinary team approach with a primary care provider, clinical pharmacist, and a dietician, patients still struggled, like there was a piece of the puzzle missing. I continued on my journey and earned my board certification in ambulatory care (BCACP), then certification as a diabetes educator (CDE, now CDCES). As time passed and I gained experience, I became more adept with dietary recommendations and motivational interviewing. I felt increasingly comfortable having lifestyle discussions with patients, which evolved over time into longer discussions in regards to goal setting and behavioral change. I worked with other multidisciplinary patient care teams with even more disciplines involved. We certainly made progress with patients, but I now recognize how much more successful patients could be if they all had a health coach.

I have been in practice as a clinical pharmacist for 16 years. While I do feel I make a difference, I am frustrated that I am seeing patients close to the point of no return. I find myself tasked with helping some of the sickest patients, often decades into chronic illness with no real way out given the damage already done to their bodies. Few have hope of ever coming off all of their current medications without radical lifestyle changes. Time and time again, I see patients start a medication to treat a symptom or side effect being caused by another drug they were previously prescribed. The cycle can continue multiple times for some patients, until they are on so many medications that they accept that drugs are the only answer. Sadly, I often find myself pondering – if someone had provided them the tools they needed 10 or 20 years ago to avoid this, would they have chosen that path? Some may have, but others, even to this day, don't have any desire to change. They would rather die an early death doing what they want, even if that means their lifestyle choices are the cause. In this free nation, people have every right to choose that fate for themselves, but I for one want to help those who don't choose that path. I want to be here for those who want to choose their health on all levels, and want to enjoy a long, healthy life, hopefully disease-free, where they can enjoy their retirement years free of constant trips to the doctor and the pharmacy for lifestyle-related illnesses that may have been prevented.

This belief that I have so much more to give is probably what led me to pursue a certification in health coaching. The more I read and learn about wellness, the more I want to read and learn about wellness. It has become a passion of mine, and it feels good to feel good. It's even more rewarding when you can help others experience the same.

If you had asked me 10 years ago what I thought about holistic wellness, I probably would have looked at you with a puzzled expression and asked, "You mean yoga and meditation?" Now I recognize the countless modalities holistic wellness encompasses and the endless possibilities for growth and improvement in mind, body, and spirit. As I continue to grow on my journey, I know my abilities and offerings will expand with me, and I for one am looking forward to being able to help people feel better on all levels.

Through my own experiences, I've found that wellness is not given, it is EARNED. The mission of my company, WELLNESS EARNED, LLC, is to help guide clients to this state, whatever that may be for them. I can help clients in multiple ways.

As an ADAPT Certified Functional Health Coach (A-CFHC), I have honed my skills to help guide clients in exploring their wellness vision to evoke their "why." Health coaching is like a dance, and the coach and client are partners. As a health coach, I aim to empower clients to take ownership of their health and wellness while offering acceptance, support, and accountability, as well as addressing challenges and blindspots along the way, All the while honoring a client-centered approach to foster possibilities and facilitate change based on the client's agenda.

As a Root Cause Protocol Consultant (RCPC), I can educate clients on their HTMA results and changes to consider to help bring the body back into balance. My hope is that the clients I work with will take their journey at their pace, using as many modalities as appropriate to get them where they want to be.

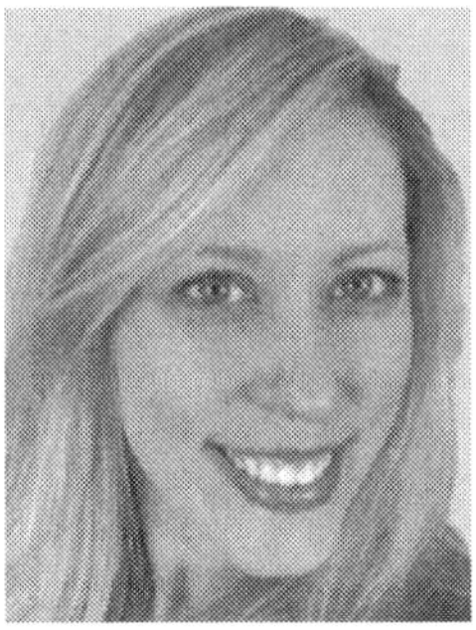

ABOUT DR. ALAINA OLENIK,

PHARMD, BCACP, CDCES, CPP, RCPC, A-CFHC, CSWWC

Dr. Alaina Olenik is a seeker of truth with a passion for learning. Her enthusiasm for all things wellness is contagious. She has spent the last 16 years working with patients managing chronic illnesses as a clinical pharmacist. She has helped hundreds of patients improve their health and has come to realize some of the limitations of conventional medicine.

In her pursuit for answers to help herself and others in a more holistic way, she became an ADAPT Certified Functional Health Coach and a Root Cause Protocol Consultant. She will also soon be a Certified STORRIE Wholistic Wellness Coach™ (CSWWC) from the STORRIE Institute™. Her genuine curiosity and ability to connect paired with her active listening skills make her an unstoppable force as a health coach. She's someone you want on your team.

As a wellness enthusiast and entrepreneur, she started her own business WELLNESS EARNED, LLC. She helps tired, stressed-out, busy individuals improve their energy and work toward their wellness vision.

She believes everyone deserves a good listening to, and seeks to do just that with all her clients.

www.wellnessearned.co | alaina.olenik@wellnessearned.co | IG: @dralainaolenik

A HEALING THAT LEAVES NO SICKNESS BEHIND

By: Dr. Zanab Qureshi,
PHARMD, CFMP, CSWWC

"O mankind, there has come to you instruction from your Lord and a healing for (the diseases) in your hearts and guidance and mercy for the believers."

– HOLY QURAN 10:57

"All disease begins in the gut."

– HIPPOCRATES

Did you know that you have a second brain? And that it's located inside of your gut? It is what causes you to feel intense emotions like having butterflies when you're excited or nervous, and feeling sick to your stomach when you're scared or emotional. This second brain is called the enteric nervous system. The enteric nervous system is made up of two thin layers that contain around 200 to 600 neurons. These neurons are nerve cells that line your gastrointestinal tract, running from your esophagus all the way down to your rectum. The second brain in your gut, or the enteric nervous system, communicates directly with the brain in your head. This is called the gut-brain connection.

I still remember the day clearly. It was a Monday morning. "Buzz buzz buzz" SNOOZE! Five minutes later, "Buzz buzz buzz." I had pressed snooze five times already. Intense fatigue had me dreading the mornings. No matter how early I went to bed, I woke up feeling drained, like I was hit by a truck. I finally got up, brushed my teeth, and got dressed for the day. It was a typical morning, always running late and grabbing breakfast on the run to class. I would get my usual: a tall iced caramel latte with whipped cream on top and a cheese Danish. The walk to my classroom building felt miles long; I would be out of breath by the time I sat at my desk. Despite drinking caffeine, it was hard concentrating during class – sometimes I would fall asleep! Although the coffee did help me get some work done, it came with its own bad side effects: stomach-wrenching pain, intestinal cramps, a jittery body, and a fast heartbeat. This kept on for six years while I pursued a Doctorate in Pharmacy.

I was in the 6th grade when my fellow classmate asked what I wished to be when I grew up. I proudly answered, "I will be a pharmacist." My choice of career was chosen for me from a young age. I never really got a chance to explore other options. I did, however, have an interest in science, particularly the human body, and I was good at math. So, I grew up dreaming that I would become a pharmacist and have extensive knowledge. I dreamt of being able to speak about illnesses and treatments confidently. I remember during the first year of pharmacy school, the university dean made each student write a letter on why they chose pharmacy as a career path. I had written that I was passionate about learning about the human body and how to use medications to treat illnesses. Most of the other college students wrote about how they would be able to start making a six-figure salary right after graduation. I however was simply very happy that I would have the privilege to help sick patients with my skills and empathy.

I am not sure if most people know how difficult and stressful pharmacy school really is. Most pharmacists study six-plus years to earn their doctorate, which includes many classes such as organic chemistry, biochemistry, anatomy & physiology, pharmacology, pathology, immunology, pharmaceutics, law, patient communication and empathy skills, simulation labs, compounding, therapeutics, and so much more! We learned over 200 drugs (specific to each body system) per month in such fine detail, with no break in between. Whew! Just writing about it gives me anxiety. This was only a part of the stress I was dealing with at the time. Having to deal with some sick family members was a whole different stress. My mind and body had gotten detrimentally affected. From the second year of pharmacy school, I started having very bad mouth and tongue ulcers. My stomach would hurt so much, twisting and burning pain. I would have a low appetite, and crave sugar, junk, and carbs. On top of my stomach ache, I would suffer from constipation and bloating!

I started visiting many different doctors to figure out what was going on. My primary care physician ran multiple blood tests – CBC, thyroid panel, lipid panel, glucose, etc. – but they would all come back normal. She referred me out to a gastroenterologist, who decided that the first thing to do was an invasive endoscopy test. I didn't have symptoms of a bleed, but for some reason the gastroenterologist felt that was the best test to do first. It was my first time getting a procedure done where they give you anesthesia. I was so nervous, and felt this was unnecessary as I was young. However, I decided to go with it, and hoped we could figure out what was wrong and treat it quickly! It was around a 30-minute procedure, and I remember when the anesthesia wore off, I thought the nurse was my mom who was trying to wake me up for school. I was insisting that I needed five more minutes of sleep. The waiting for results was quite nerve-wrecking, however the reports came back normal. I was relieved that it was not a big illness. The gastroenterologist was quite confused as well. She didn't run any other tests, and she did not ask about my diet, stressors, or sleep. She gave me a prescription for omeprazole, a proton pump inhibitor to reduce the acid in my stomach. When I went back for a follow-up three months later, she wanted me to continue taking the medication because I felt a little better.

Although the acid reflux was a little better, I still felt extremely fatigued, and was getting mouth sores on the sides of my tongue. So, I decided to visit a dentist and have my teeth evaluated, thinking maybe they are hitting the sides of my tongue while I sleep. She ran some X-rays and said, "I see no issues, your teeth are perfectly aligned." She suggested that I avoid eating spicy foods for the time being to allow my tongue to heal. That was quite upsetting, as I come from a Desi background, and our food is filled with different spices. My mom would cook separate bland food just for me. Bland food was not fun, however it did help with my tongue sores. Anytime I felt the food was slightly spicy, I would get so paranoid that I would develop tongue sores again. It really affected my quality of life. I started sticking to specific routines, extremely afraid that any change would bring about all the symptoms and pain again, and I continued taking omeprazole for a couple of years.

After graduating from pharmacy school, I was so happy with my big accomplishment. Even before my graduation, I got a job offer to work at a big chain community pharmacy. Pharmacy interns who were working longer than I was did not get the job offer. My pharmacy manager told me that I was given preference due to my strong passion and knowledge for counseling patients. Throughout my internship, I never let any opportunity go where I did not teach a patient something about their health or the medication they were picking up. It felt very fulfilling to have conversations with and be of some benefit for people who were looking to feel better. I would provide words of encouragement and pointers on how to better adhere to the medication they were prescribed. As a community pharmacist, I continued this passion and work ethic. But, I soon realized that the managers would not be happy when I spent extra time with patients. They just wanted the prescriptions to be filled fast for more business. If I spent time with patients, the lines would get long and work would get backed up. To my surprise and despite all my efforts, it was impossible to provide quality personalized care and fill the prescriptions, answer doctor calls, help the drive-thru line, and finish my shift on time. Accuracy and patient care was not as important as they advertised to the customers. We were told that the numbers were the most important. Corporate bosses wanted to see high prescription fill and vaccination numbers.

Despite my disappointment, I continued working long hours with no breaks. Community pharmacists are expected to stand for 10-12 hours continuously without getting a chance to eat or use the bathroom. I would come home late feeling extremely exhausted, eat dinner at 11 p.m., pop a Tums, and scroll on my phone until I fell asleep. In the morning, it was the same thing all over again. I would run out, grab coffee and some sugary breakfast, then crash by lunch time. Most of the time I would miss lunch if we were not caught up on prescriptions, or if I had a little bit of time, I would inhale my lunch in five minutes so I could get back to work. My quality of life and health were deteriorating. I started feeling severe stomach and intestinal pains again, like there was a hole in my stomach.

Soon, my dream job started to feel unfulfilling, and I felt the symptoms all over again, even more intense than the last time. I decided that this time I would visit a different gastroenterologist, hoping she would give me a better diagnosis. When I explained my symptoms – stomach-wrenching pain, bloating, constipation, acid reflux, fatigue, nausea, headaches – she decided to do an emergency endoscopy. She said, "I need to see what is going on inside and rule out anything major." To her surprise, the endoscopy came back normal, so she decided to order a CT scan, which also came back normal. At that point, she was confused and told me to take Nexium (another proton pump inhibitor) for a few weeks and then start taking famotidine. But, I knew the medications weren't fixing the problem, so I asked her to run some other tests. We tested for H-pylori, which also came back negative.

I was so frustrated and felt hopeless. I decided to keep a log of which foods were causing the symptoms, and noticed that soda, tomato sauce, coffee, and spicy foods were on the top of my list. So, I decided to avoid those foods. At this point, I had paranoia about any food I ate. I would not like to eat out, afraid that something would trigger the pain. I also decided to expand my pharmacy experience, so I joined an inpatient hospital pharmacy as a part-time pharmacist. I hoped that maybe I could be of a better benefit and create a healthier lifestyle. But, it was extremely tough balancing both jobs, personal life, and my worsening health.

Then the unimaginable happened: a pandemic hit and made the workload even more strenuous. Healthcare workers got the most affected, working even longer hours all whilst wearing protective gear. My anxiety and stress was off the charts. At this point, the fatigue was unbearable – constant headaches that no Tylenol or Excedrin would relieve, stomach pains that each food would provoke. I couldn't take it anymore! I had to take a break, so I decided to go on a work leave.

During my break, I kept working at the hospital. But, I was determined to feel better. I was tired of going to doctors who would say there was nothing wrong with me. All the labs would come back fine, but I still felt very sick. No one could understand how bad the fatigue was and how every food gave me anxiety because I would be scared of intense stomach pains that would come about. I started to research, and spent hours reading healthcare articles and watching videos. One day I came across a naturopath. She specialized in natural healing for chronic issues like irritable bowel syndrome, anxiety, depression, polycystic ovary syndrome, thyroid issues, insulin resistance, weight loss, infertility, chronic pain, fatigue, etc.

Finally, I felt hope again. The light at the end of the tunnel seemed a lot closer. My visit with her was so refreshing, I finally felt heard and understood. I wasn't crazy – my body was actually getting sick and the symptoms I felt were real. She went over everything at my appointment, which was over one hour long and every aspect was discussed – emotional health, spiritual well-being, diet/nutrition, sleep hygiene, menstrual cycle, and my stressors. I couldn't believe how everything was so connected, and when one goes bad the rest follows shortly after. She recommended some Functional Medicine testing that came back to show I had adrenal dysfunction, inflammation in the gut, imbalanced gut microbiome, and mildly low thyroid function. She could tell all of this by a simple minerals, hormone, and gut test. Her treatment plan was very simple and tailored to fit my specific lifestyle and needs. This personalized care allowed me to follow and adhere to our plan easily. In her treatment plan, we focused on improving sleep hygiene, mindful breathing and eating, positive affirmations, aromatherapy, and supplements for adrenal and thyroid support. After the first appointment, we planned a follow-up in three months to start working on rebuilding gut health.

I had mentioned to my naturopath that in my clinical experience as a pharmacist, I came to realize that most medications for chronic issues were being used as a bandage to mask the symptoms and not address the root cause. Although I believe that conventional Western medicine has its place, especially in acute illnesses, I was still very fascinated that Functional Medicine was the missing puzzle piece in healthcare, especially for preventative care and to help heal chronic illnesses. She recommended that I specialize in Functional Medicine, and use it with the passion I had when I first started pharmacy school to help patients who were suffering like I was.

Functional Medicine is a systems biology–based approach that focuses on identifying and addressing the root cause of disease. Each symptom is in fact interconnected. And in my case, the damaged gut-brain connection was contributing to many of the symptoms.

You see, the gut-brain connection is what causes you to feel things like a fight-or-flight response and nervousness before giving a presentation. Many people deal with other conditions that affect their physical and gut health. If you feel things like anxiety or depression, this can cause intestinal distress, causing problems in the stomach or bowels. Because of the gut-brain connection, the reverse can also be true – your gut health affects your mental and physical health.

Your enteric nervous system can impact your emotions. In turn, your emotions can have an effect on certain conditions, like:

- Irritable bowel syndrome (IBS)
- Constipation
- Bloating
- Pain
- Diarrhea
- Stomach aches

While conventional medicine diagnoses and treats what's above the surface (symptoms and disease), Functional Medicine also looks at what's below the surface, at the root of the disease, such as environmental and lifestyle factors, including sleep and relaxation, physical activity (exercise), nutrition, stress, relationships, toxins, and water.

During my leave, not only did I learn how to improve my physical health, I also focused on my spiritual healing. I had a lot going on with very little support. Turning my focus toward God and my religion helped me from losing hope. I started to study Islam in depth. Although I was born Muslim, there was so much in the holy book Quran and from the teachings of the Prophet Muhammad (peace be upon him) that I didn't know.

I came to realize that Functional Medicine was not new, and was actually practiced in a similar manner many many years ago. Over 1400 years ago, religious scriptures taught civilization the best way to eat, drink, sleep, pray, etc., all of which is being confirmed by science today. An example would be that the Prophet Muhammad (peace be upon him) had said, *"The son of Adam does not fill any vessel worse than his stomach. It is enough for the son of Adam to eat a few mouthfuls to straighten his back, but if he must (fill his stomach), then one third for his food, one third for his drink, and one third for his breath."* Today, science researchers agree that restricted calorie intake may prolong a healthy life by preventing age-related illnesses. Also, every year in the Holy month of Ramadan, Muslims all over the world complete fast (no food and no water) from dawn to sunset for 30 days. Today, science has shown tremendous benefits for fasting, such as restoring homeostasis in the body by helping take out the cellular garbage and reducing inflammatory markers.

I also started to study prophetic medicine known as *Tibb-e-Nabvi.* This is the knowledge of medicine practiced by the Prophet Muhammad (peace be upon him) to cure illnesses of the body, mind, and spirit. This includes the modern practice of "food is medicine" and viewing the body as a whole when treating a patient.

In Islam, we have a prayer that is asked when you or someone is sick. This prayer is, "*O Allah, Lord of mankind, do away with my suffering. Heal (me) as You are the only Healer and there is no cure except that of Yours,* ***it is that which leaves no sickness behind.***" This prayer has become my motto; I have a vision to help patients to heal from within, to help bring back the body's natural homeostasis, to heal all aspects – the mind, body, and soul. The expertise that I gained from studying this aspect of medicine has only grown my passion. And now, I want to share my knowledge, experience, and passion with the world.

Therefore, I created my company, Afiyah Wellbeing, a healthcare center that is inspired by natural healing and prophetic medicine. The word *Afiyah* is very close to my heart. What is Afiyah you may ask? It is the shortest most powerful prayer. It is reported that more than 1400 years ago, a person named Al Abbas came to the Prophet Muhammad (peace be upon him) and said, "Teach me something to ask God Almighty." The Prophet (peace be upon him) said, "Ask God for *Afiyah (Wellness).*" [Tirmidhi 3514].

Do you know what Afiyah is?

To be saved from any affliction, you are in Afiyah.

To be healthy, you are in Afiyah.

To have enough money, you are in Afiyah.

To live, you are in Afiyah.

To have your children protected, you are in Afiyah.

So in short, Afiyah is wellness. But this isn't just any kind of wellness; it's a complete wellness. I'm sure that everyone's dream is to be free from any illness, grief, distress, hardship, harm, and financial issues.

The Prophet (peace be upon him) said, "There are two blessings which many people do not appreciate: health and leisure." In today's time, we do not value or take care of our health nor free time. We need to aim for a work-life balance. Don't exert yourself, and moderation in whatever you do is a necessity. With the right guidance and support, you can transform your life. I am here to tell you, there is still hope and I can help you. Give yourself permission to heal, a chance to change for the better, and a chance to change your life around.

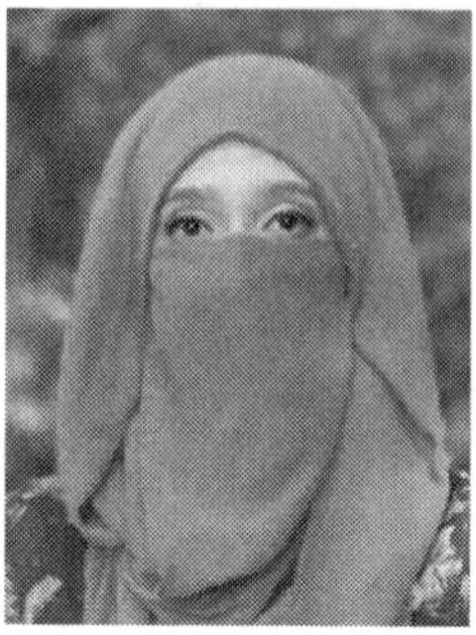

ABOUT DR. ZANAB QURESHI,

PHARMD, CFMP, CSWWC

Dr. Zanab Qureshi has completed her degree in Doctor of Pharmacy. She has worked in both acute and chronic settings as a hospital and community pharmacist. She is privileged to work closely with a variety of different interpersonal teams in healthcare including oncology. As a clinical pharmacist, she has extensive knowledge about planning medication interventions, caring for patients, and optimizing therapy choices. Her expertise in dosages and customization of care plans has allowed her to be successful at educating patients and improving physician knowledge to maximize treatment success.

Dr. Zanab is also a Certified Functional Medicine Practitioner (CFMP) and Integrative Pharmacy Health Specialist, a Certified STORRIE Wholistic Wellness Coach™(CSWWC), and an Islamic Educator for women and kids. She is the creator of Afiyah Wellbeing, a healthcare center inspired by Prophetic and Natural Healing.

She is kind-hearted, passion-driven, and extremely empathic. She loves counseling and helping patients feel better by empowering and guiding them. After her own personal health journey, she is passionate about helping women get back their energy by optimizing gut health and guiding them on stress management. She utilizes natural therapy with a strong focus on a whole-body approach. Her programs aim to balance the mind, body, and soul.

www.afiyahwellbeing.com | info@afiyahwellbeing.com |
IG: @afiyahwellbeing

EMBRACING MINDFULNESS: A JOURNEY TOWARD BALANCE, WELL-BEING, AND PURPOSE

By: Dr. Nhu Truong,
PHARMD

"In a fast-paced world, where burnout and exhaustion prevail, it's time to pause, reflect, and find solace in the present moment. Join me on a transformative journey toward mindfulness, intention, and purpose."

– Dr. Nhu Truong

Living in a fast-paced, materialistic world, we often neglect our own well-being. Yet, to truly care for others, we must prioritize our physical, mental, and spiritual health. As a healthcare professional with over 13 years of experience, I emphasize the importance of taking responsibility for our own well-being. While medication has its place, preventing illness through self-care and a holistic approach is crucial. Self-love, mindfulness, and daily meditation have helped me reduce stress and improve my overall health. (Mindfulness is defined as a mental state achieved by focusing one's awareness on the present moment, while calmly acknowledging and accepting one's feelings, thoughts, and bodily sensations, used as a therapeutic technique.)

In this chapter, I share my personal journey of self-discovery and transformation amidst the challenges and changes brought about by the COVID-19 pandemic. As a busy, working mom and entrepreneur, I am constantly striving to excel in my professional life while ensuring the well-being of my family. However, this relentless pursuit led to burnout and a neglect of my own self-care. Through the tragic loss of a loved one and my subsequent exploration of mindfulness meditation, I learned valuable lessons about the importance of balance, self-love, and finding purpose in life.

Before the pandemic, I was a dedicated mom, juggling a demanding full-time job as the Director of Clinical Services and pursuing my own e-commerce venture in the health and wellness industry. However, the weight of my responsibilities, combined with neglecting self-care, left me mentally and physically exhausted. It took a toll on my well-being, leading to high blood pressure and a sense of burnout.

I had always prioritized others, emulating the selflessness I learned from my mother. However, in doing so, I neglected myself. It wasn't until I experienced the tragic loss of my beloved nephew during the COVID-19 pandemic that my perspective shifted, urging me to seek a path of self-discovery, personal growth, and well-being.

"Adaptability is not about resisting change; it's about embracing it and finding new opportunities within it."

– SIMON SINEK

The COVID-19 pandemic presented unprecedented challenges for individuals and businesses alike. While some struggled to adapt, others found opportunities for innovation and growth. The importance of having a backup plan and/or side gig became apparent as the future became uncertain. Traits like adaptability, perseverance, and grit became essential for navigating this changing landscape.

Amidst the pandemic, I learned firsthand about the stark reality of mental health issues and the profound impact they can have. Witnessing the loss of loved ones to COVID-19 and suicide heightened my awareness, and it was a wake-up call that prompted me to reflect on what truly matters in life.

"Putting yourself first is not selfish. It's necessary for self-care and overall well-being."
– Oprah Winfrey

My previous mindset of prioritizing work and others above all else proved detrimental to my own well-being. It was crucial for me to acknowledge the signs of burnout resulting in high blood pressure, which I had ignored for far too long. It took the wise words of my husband to make me realize that I was neglecting my own health and happiness in pursuit of success in my career. I witnessed firsthand the impact of stress on my well-being, and I knew it was time to make a change NOW. I learned the importance of putting my health and family first.

"Meditation is not an escape from reality; it is an entry into the fullness of reality."
– Jon Kabat-Zinn

The pandemic shed light on the prevalence of mental health issues, including anxiety and depression. Tragically, I experienced the loss of a loved one to suicide, which deeply affected my perspective on life's priorities. Through practicing mindfulness meditation, I discovered the power of calming the mind and cultivating inner peace. This chapter now explores the profound impact of mindfulness on mental health and well-being.

"Mindfulness is the key to unlocking the full potential of your mind, body, and spirit."
– Deepak Chopra

Discovering mindfulness meditation became a turning point in my journey. Learning from my teacher, Lama Nawang Kunphel, I realized that mindfulness is essential for everyone, regardless of their religious and/or spiritual beliefs. By cultivating mindfulness in our thoughts, speech, and actions, we can create a positive impact on ourselves and those around us. Mindfulness allows us to be fully present in each moment, fostering gratitude, kindness, and compassion toward ourselves and others. This newfound mindfulness in my daily life practice brought calmness, reduced stress, and helped me gain clarity on what truly matters in life.

Embracing Impermanence, Gratitude, and Finding Inner Peace

"The most powerful meditation is the meditation on impermanence."
– Dalai Lama

The heart-breaking loss of my nephew emphasized the impermanence of life, reminding us that tomorrow is never guaranteed, and we need to cherish every waking moment in our lives. The experience compelled me to prioritize my well-being and seek inner peace. Mindfulness meditation became a transformative tool, enabling me to shift my mindset and find calm amidst chaos.

Practicing gratitude and embracing the present became vital habits of my everyday life. By recognizing the value of time and the importance of self-care, I learned to lead a more fulfilling and purposeful life.

"Your purpose in life is to find your purpose and give your whole heart and soul to it."

– BUDDHA

Reflecting on my diverse career path, I have always yearned for a more meaningful and fulfilling purpose on this planet. Growing up as a little girl, I always questioned the purpose of life. It seemed like a mere cycle of birth, growing up, going to school, starting a family, having kids, becoming grandparents, growing old, and eventually dying. I often pondered on and questioned this cycle, as well as desired to do something different and not fall into the same path as everyone else. I have always wanted to help others, make an impact on the world, and serve others.

My family immigrated to the United States, which is considered the land of the free and full of opportunities, from Vietnam when I was around 10 years old. My parents made the decision to leave everything behind, including their friends, family, and home, in pursuit of a better education, greater opportunities, and freedom for their children. I am eternally grateful for my parents' unconditional love and sacrifices, which have provided me and my siblings with a better life. I am forever thankful to be in this country in which we are given the opportunity to better ourselves, thrive, and give back to the community.

While growing up, I aspired to be a teacher or a doctor, which led me to pursue a career in the pharmaceutical/healthcare industry. However, through my experiences and observations, I have come to realize that in order to bring about the changes we want to see in our current healthcare system, we must be the catalysts for change. We cannot expect others to change or attempt to change others if they are not ready to change themselves. It all starts within us.

I consider myself fortunate to have witnessed my older sister's health journey and how our family embraced a holistic approach to treat her asthma/COPD, even when we were still in Vietnam. Our exploration of natural remedies and determination to find a cure left a lasting impression on me. Recently, my younger sister was diagnosed with diabetes, which can be attributed to the constant stress of her high-pressure corporate job as a Senior Vice President in a top investment banking firm. While she is taking medication for her diabetes, she has also incorporated holistic lifestyle modifications, such as adopting healthier eating habits and incorporating bitter melon into her diet to help lower her blood sugar levels.

I experienced my own health crisis when I was admitted to the hospital with sepsis due to stress and burnout. The thought of leaving behind my family and young children terrified me. They have always served as my motivation and wake-up call, reminding me why I am driven to help others thrive and live life on their own terms. Prioritizing my children and family became a defining factor, reinforcing the importance of being present in their lives. My journey toward health and well-being continues, with mindfulness at the core of how I relate to myself and others.

"Your habits shape your identity, and your identity shapes your habits."
– James Clear

Through my experiences, I have witnessed a recurring theme among business owners, doctors, pharmacists and other healthcare providers who have lost sight of the human side of their professions. Many lack empathy and compassion for one another when faced with challenging situations, such as car breakdowns, sick children, or their own personal health struggles. It is disheartening to see managers, bosses, or owners who do not genuinely care for their patients, clients, or employees and speak negatively about them behind their backs. They exhibit poor work ethic, engage in micromanagement, show disrespect toward their employees, and may even resort to verbal abuse or threats of termination. This realization became a turning point for me, as I could no longer work for or serve under individuals who lacked moral and ethical values. It goes against everything I stand for and does not align with my core principles. Prior to deciding to leave my last position, I had a heartfelt conversation with my co-worker, assuring her that it was okay for me to leave and encouraging her to stay until she found another job for financial stability.

During that conversation, my co-worker became emotional and shared her recent journey of returning to the workforce, specifically in pharmacy, after completing rehab for a drug overdose. Her attempt to end her life was a result of burnout and the toxic environment created by a demanding manager at a busy store where she worked full-time. Initially, she believed that transitioning to part-time hours at our workplace would be manageable. However, she confided that the only reason she stayed was because of me. She was amazed that, regardless of how poorly the owner or manager behaved, I remained steadfast and composed. She witnessed firsthand my genuine care for her and our patients/customers as I consistently went above and beyond to meet their needs. This experience emphasized the profound impact we can have on someone else's life. Our words and actions can alter the trajectory of their lives.

There is another employee at our workplace who joined us for their first job and remains unaware that a better world awaits them. I empathize with those who feel trapped in toxic environments due to financial obligations or fear of negative repercussions. These stories serve as a reminder that we never truly know what someone else is going through in their life outside of work. Therefore, it is crucial to offer grace, give people chances, listen attentively, and show empathy towards our employees, co-workers, and customers. When we genuinely care for others and prioritize their best interests, we can make a positive difference in their lives. It is important to let them know that there are people out there who care, support, and uplift them instead of abusing them.

It is always wise to have a backup plan or financial cushion in case a company unexpectedly shuts down or if you need to leave your job for the sake of your mental well-being. No amount of money is worth being stuck in a place where you are treated poorly, where mutual respect is lacking, where professional licenses are compromised, or where ethical boundaries are crossed. Remember that things happen for a reason. Have confidence in yourself and stand by your values. If prayer and manifestation resonate with you, trust in their power and believe that the universe will deliver at the right time. Trust your intuition.

"Time does not wait for anyone, therefore, the time to seek your own purpose is now. We need to ask ourselves, 'Are you living your life with joy and happiness?'"

– Dr. Nhu Truong

"Failure is success in progress."

– Albert Einstein

Failure is not a roadblock, but a stepping stone toward growth. Embracing failure allows us to re-evaluate, learn from experiences, and come back even stronger. Comparison with others is futile, as everyone has their unique journey and own timing. By comparing myself less to others and focusing on my own progress, I gained a sense of empowerment and confidence. By working diligently and becoming the best version of ourselves, we pave the way for success and contribute positively to the lives of others.

My Mission Statement

In a world desperately in need of mindfulness and purpose, I am dedicated to empowering and inspiring burnt-out professionals to regain control of their lives. Through embracing mindfulness, intention, and purpose, we can create thriving businesses and find joy and happiness in the present moment. Together, we can nurture a community that cherishes well-being, uplifts one another, and embraces the beauty of life.

My Vision Statement

My vision is for individuals of all ages to embrace mindfulness daily, fostering well-being in our families, communities, and the world we call home.

Mindfulness is a powerful tool that can transform our lives and help us thrive in the face of challenges. By prioritizing self-care, adopting a mindful approach to daily living, and embracing impermanence, we can find joy, fulfillment, and purpose. Remember, you are responsible for your own well-being, and through mindfulness, you can create a life that aligns with your deepest values and aspirations.

By incorporating mindfulness into our lives, we can find inner peace, balance, and purpose. Embracing change, prioritizing self-care, and being present in each moment can lead to a more fulfilling and joyful existence. I invite you to embark on your own mindfulness journey, recognizing that we all have unique gifts to share with the world. Together, we can create a more mindful and compassionate society.

My Gratitude Statement

I am profoundly grateful for all the people and experiences that have helped shape my life, especially during the most difficult and challenging times. My heartfelt gratitude goes out to my friends, parents, relatives, co-workers/colleagues, bosses, and teachers who have supported and guided me to become the person I am today. Without their influence, I would be nothing.

In particular, I am immensely thankful for my loving and compassionate teacher, Lama Nawang Kunphel. He has shown me the importance of having aspirations to help others and alleviate their suffering. He has taught me to extend love and compassion to all beings as if they were my own family. With his wisdom and knowledge, he has inspired me to believe that our impact on the world is boundless.

May we all strive to be a guiding light in the lives of those who need our support. May our actions be the catalyst for the happiness and well-being of others.

As you reach the end of this chapter, remember this: the power to transform your burnout into purpose-driven success is within your grasp. You are not defined by exhaustion; you are defined by your capacity to rise.

Imagine a life where your passion burns brighter than ever, where resilience guides you through every challenge, and mindfulness becomes the foundation of your decisions. Envision a business that not only survives but thrives, powered by innovative strategies and a renewed sense of purpose. Picture yourself living a life that resonates with joy and accomplishment, a life that's fully aligned with your aspirations.

The call to action is clear. Don't let burnout be the final chapter of your story. Join our community of burnout conquerors and determined entrepreneurs who are actively reshaping their lives. Embrace change as your ally, and together, we will rewrite the script of exhaustion, replacing it with a symphony of energy, passion, and brilliance.

Let's embark on this path of growth and renewal together. Your brighter future begins with a choice and a commitment to your well-being and success. Here's to unlocking your full potential and igniting a life of purpose, joy, and achievement. The journey starts now.

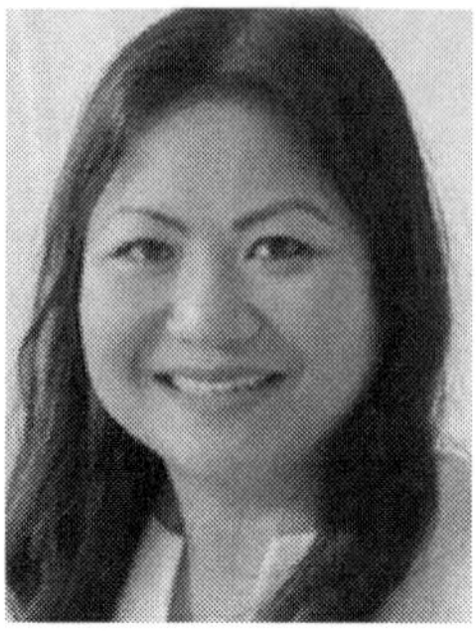

ABOUT DR. NHU TRUONG,
PHARMD

Introducing a Transformative Journey to Empowerment and Mindful Living. Embark on a profound journey of self-discovery and empowerment with Dr. Nhu Truong, a seasoned Functional Medicine/Holistic Practitioner, STORRIE™ Ambassador, and a dedicated member of the BURN OUT TO ALL OUT team. With over 23 years of industry expertise, Dr. Truong's remarkable path from Clinical Pharmacist to thriving entrepreneur is an inspiring testament to the transformative power of awareness and mindfulness meditation.

Dr. Truong's personal evolution from a super-working mom entrenched in Corporate America, to a holistic visionary championing well-being, offers a compelling narrative of resilience and change. The pivotal moment of her own burnout, a distressing encounter that led her to hospitalization due to stress-induced sepsis, ignited her purpose. Through unwavering determination, she reclaimed her physical and mental well-being, shattering the chains of pharmaceutical dependence through holistic living.

At the heart of Dr. Truong's calling lies her profound commitment to guide others towards their health aspirations. Infused with mindfulness and meditation, she empowers individuals to incorporate small, meaningful changes into their daily lives, leading to remarkable transformations. By fostering a culture of intention and purpose, reinforced by compassion, kindness, and love, she propels burnout professionals and entrepreneurs to soar to new heights of well-being.

In her role as advocate, mentor, and business development partner, Dr. Truong is dedicated to enriching your journey. Her affinity for like-minded entrepreneurs, driven by a shared vision of serving their communities while addressing mental health and burnout, cultivates a thriving ecosystem of support. With a diverse background spanning clinical expertise, sales, and management, she is uniquely positioned to guide and champion your growth.

Dr. Truong's keen belief in the innate human potential to overcome adversity and ignite change resonates deeply. She's committed to reshaping lives through mentoring, and inspiring those struggling with the relentless demands of work, family, and health. Her mission extends beyond empowerment; it is a rallying cry for embracing the present moment, finding happiness, and nurturing gratitude regardless of life's challenges.

Dr. Truong passionately asserts that every individual possesses a unique gift, waiting to be unveiled through mindful meditation. She encapsulates the profound notion that genuine joy and abundance spring from within, forming the bedrock of a life well-lived.

Join Dr. Nhu Truong on a journey of transformation, where empowerment, mindfulness, and purpose converge to create a tapestry of wellness, prosperity, and boundless gratitude. Let her guide you in unlocking your true potential and crafting a life that radiates positivity and fulfillment. Connect with Dr. Truong today to embark on a life-changing partnership and uncover the infinite possibilities that await.

www.knhealthconsulting.com | nhu@knhealthconsulting.com |
LI: @drnhutruong

IN ORDER TO HEAL, YOU MUST CHANGE

By: Michelle Thompson,
PA, FMP, CSWWC

"If you always do what you've always done, you'll always get what you always got."
– Henry Ford

I knew when I was 6 years old, I was going to be a nurse. My mother was a nurse, my father and grandfather were firefighters. They were my heroes – taking care and "fixing"everyone.

After I finished nursing school, I always worked two jobs at the same time. I worked in a hospital and in an outpatient clinic so I could work in a variety of settings. I went from working in an oncology unit to labor and delivery/nursery – two completely different realms because I loved everything in every area.

Fast forward to marrying my high school sweetheart, who also became a firefighter, to having four beautiful girls whom I adore.

When my oldest daughter was 12 years old and my youngest daughter was 5 weeks old, my oldest daughter was diagnosed with a tennis ball-sized brain mass. She was life-flighted for emergency craniotomy (brain surgery). They told me she'd never walk, talk, or be able to take care of herself again. Our local pediatric neurologist said I would need to put her in a nursing home and I would never be able to take care of her. I was devastated! I had a 1-month-old and a 14-month-old at home, and my other daughter was 8. My firefighter husband worked an average of 100 hours a week, and also worked at another job on the side, so he was never home. How was I going to help my daughter learn how to walk again, how to feed herself, how to get dressed and bathe independently with a newborn and a one-year-old and an 8-year-old. I could do it! We could do it! We just needed to believe we could do anything if we put our minds to it. With God's help, and a strong belief, I knew we would win this battle. I could keep my daughter out of the nursing home.

After years of physical therapy, occupational therapy, and speech therapy to help improve strength and coordination, we started to see improvement. Weekly hospital visits for IVIG treatments, which was an experimental treatment because there was no known treatment for myelinoclastic diffuse sclerosis. She was in case studies around the world and in medical journals, because her disease was so rare. I was determined to fight this battle with her! Long story, short, we won. She won! She did NOT end up in a nursing home like her local neurologist told us! She learned how to walk again, how to feed herself, and become more independent. I had slept an average of five hours per night for several years since I could only do research on rare neurological diseases after my four girls were asleep for the night, but it was worth it.

When physicians from all over started to call me, asking for advice and recommendations on brain tumors in children, I knew I needed to do more to help everyone! I remembered how I felt when no one could give me answers. I did not want anyone to ever feel the way I felt. I knew at that moment I could help more people if I became a provider. My love for neurology was developed. Brain health was so fascinating. A lot of diagnoses are complex, and you can't order labs and form a diagnosis immediately. After years of studying rare, neurological diseases, multiple sclerosis, etc. to help my daughter, I knew God put me here to do more, help more, give people hope if they didn't have it, be their confidence, be their cheerleader.

Before becoming a Functional Medicine practitioner, I was a physician assistant and a nurse for 25-plus years. I have worked in neurology, family practice, internal medicine, surgery, and OB/gynecology. I'm currently working in the nation's first Women's Alzheimer's Movement Prevention Center for disease prevention at Cleveland Clinic.

Forty percent of Alzheimer's disease cases are preventable with lifestyle modifications including diet, sleep, movement, stress management, and socialization. By modifying risk factors, we can decrease our chances of ending up with Alzheimer's. Two-thirds of all currently diagnosed individuals are women! Women! I currently have a three-year waiting list to get in for a personalized evaluation, so we narrowed the age group to 30-50. A lot of my patients fly in from out of state for an evaluation and fly out within 24 hours. I feel they have spent a lot of money for their commitment to disease prevention, and I am so proud of them! I always go above and beyond Alzheimer's prevention in every visit. I feel that disease prevention is important for all areas including cardiovascular, hormones, nutrition, gut health, sleep, insulin resistance, and so many other key factors.

I always say let's be proactive instead of reactive. Let's prevent everything we can from occurring instead of waiting and fixing the problem later.

I've always been passionate about helping others reach their personal version of success. Over the past 15 years, my love for Functional Medicine and holistic wellness has continued to strengthen. Finding the root cause, using food as medicine, nutraceuticals when appropriate, being proactive in preventive care, and biohacking aging is the key.

I took classes in Functional Medicine through the Institute of Functional Medicine (IFM). I completed my Comprehensive Weight Loss Management certification through the American Academy of Anti-Aging Medicine's Metabolic Medical Institute. I think it's important to continue to educate ourselves with as much training as possible. Medicine is always changing and learning must never end. We have to educate ourselves with courses, classes, fellowships, etc. I love conventional/traditional medicine, but when you only get 10 minutes to evaluate, diagnose, and treat each patient, there is not enough time. You cannot manage and reverse chronic diseases in that amount of time. We all deserve more than 10 minutes. The reason I went into medicine was to give excellent care and go that extra mile for my patients. When I started to feel that I couldn't give that kind of care, I knew it was time to focus on Functional Medicine and holistic wellness.

Today, I am working at Cleveland Clinic in a phenomenal Women's Alzheimer's Prevention Center, but I know I need to continue to give and serve even more.

I am fascinated with nutrigenomics and testing. I can provide extensive education and a customized plan for your individual genetics, based on your DNA. I can help you improve your health and overall well-being.

I would further investigate and add any other functional tests if needed, including food sensitivity, hormone health, metal toxicity or generalized toxicity, gut health, and an overall nutritional evaluation.

"The meaning of life is to find your gift.
The purpose of life is to give it away."
– Dr. Radka Toms

I can't love this quote enough. We are all here to serve. When you find your gift, give it away. I hope to educate and help thousands and thousands more.

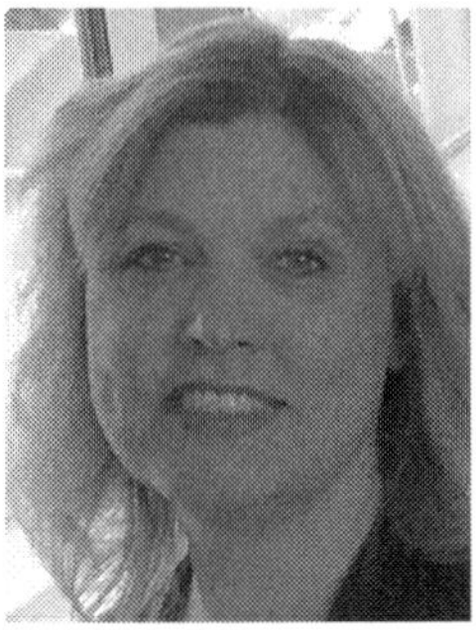

ABOUT MICHELLE THOMPSON,

PA, FMP, CSWWC

Michelle Thompson is a Physician Associate, functional medicine practitioner, wellness advocate, wife, and mother of 4 girls.

Her experience includes both inpatient and outpatient settings. She has a wide range of experience which includes: Women's health, family practice, internal medicine, surgery, Neurology, Weight loss, Wellness, and Prevention. She worked 6 years at Cleveland Clinic in cognitive disorders specializing in early onset dementia, Alzheimer's, Lewy body disease, and MS. In addition, she is currently in the process of becoming a Certified STORRIE Wholistic Wellness Coach™ (CSWWC) from STORRIE Institute™.

She worked for the last 2 years in the world's first Alzheimer's prevention center for women only at Cleveland Clinic focusing on brain health.

She has been dedicated to helping others achieve better physical and emotional well-being through dietary modifications, physical activity, sleep, and relaxation practices. She focuses on brain health, healthy lifestyle changes, and prevention while improving chronic diseases.

She focuses on all components looking for underlying causes of disease. Extra emphasis is placed on hormones, nutrition, stress, sleep, supplements, and reducing inflammation and exercise. Focusing on perimenopausal and postmenopausal women with a proven and preventive approach to overcoming hormonal imbalances. Education and clarity is the key to success.

She empowers everyone with the knowledge, information, and resources they need to not only live longer but live a healthier more fulfilled life. She helps them to focus on their goals and helps them with obstacles so they have a fulfilled fun mid-life with energy. Feeling their ultimate best self, both physically and emotionally.

Nutrition, Managing Hormones, Movement, Sleep, and Stress Modification are just a few of the essentials to achieve wellness and overall health optimization.

She remains passionate about helping you be your ultimate best self using holistic approaches to help guide you towards optimal health and long-lasting wellness.

OptimalwellnesswithMichelle@gmail.com |
IG: @Optimalwellness_withMichelle | LI: @Michelle Thompson

FROM CANCER SCARE TO FITNESS FLARE

By: Jackie Lyn Velasco,
MS, RPH

"At the end, it's not about what you have or even what you've accomplished.
It's about who you've lifted up, who you've made better.
It's about what you have given back."

– Denzel Washington

Introduction

I remember the day I received the news like it was yesterday. The doctor's voice was gentle, but the words hit me like a ton of bricks. *"I'm sorry, but the test results show that you have a tumor in your throat,"* he said. *"We need to run some more tests to determine if it is cancerous."*

My mind raced as he spoke. I thought about my three young children and my loving husband. *How would they survive without me? Who would take care of them?* The thought of leaving them behind was unbearable.

The days that followed were a blur of appointments, tests, and waiting rooms. My husband was by my side every step of the way, holding my hand and offering words of comfort. However, fear and anxiety were always there, lurking just beneath the surface.

I was devastated. I didn't want to believe it. I was angry and frustrated. Why did this have to happen to me? I was young and healthy, or so I thought. I didn't want to go through any treatment or surgery. I was scared.

Having worked as an oncology pharmacist in the past, I have witnessed firsthand the immense struggles that cancer patients endure on their journey toward recovery. I have seen the pain, the uncertainty, and the sheer strength that these individuals possess in the face of such a formidable adversary. Every day, I witnessed the devastating side effects of various treatments, and my heart went out to every patient who walked through our doors.

My role then extended beyond simply dispensing chemotherapy; I became a source of solace and support for those grappling with the physical and emotional toll of their illness. I spent countless hours counseling patients, answering their questions, and providing them with the knowledge they needed to navigate their treatment plans. I saw the fear in their eyes, the vulnerability that comes with battling a disease that knows no boundaries.

As life presented me with its own set of challenges, I found myself facing the possibility of being on the other side. The thought of undergoing the same treatments, experiencing the same side effects, and being faced with the same uncertainties that I have witnessed in my patients, filled me with a mixture of dread and empathy, not only for myself but also for my family.

As we waited for the final diagnosis, I found myself making plans for the worst-case scenario. I thought of writing letters to my children, telling them how much I loved them and how proud I was of them. I made arrangements for their care, just in case.

My family and I moved here to the United States to be able to provide a better life for them and a better future, and to provide financial help to my folks and siblings back home, which is a typical immigrant story.

During this time, I worked as a community pharmacist. Being a pharmacist was my childhood dream. I was inspired by what pharmacists do. When I was in fourth grade, I read in a science journal about a Filipino scientist named Dr. Magdalena Cantoria. She was a botanist and a pharmacist. From that article, what I learned was that pharmacists discover and compound medicines to cure people who are sick, and for me, at that time it meant those who have terminal illnesses like cancer.

I love my job as a pharmacist. Every day, I have the opportunity to make a positive impact on people's lives by ensuring they receive the right medications and healthcare advice. It's a fulfilling and rewarding profession that allows me to combine my passion for science with my desire to help others. Despite my love for my job, the environment I worked in at that time was toxic. I had been working in the same place for years, and over time, I noticed a significant workplace change. The atmosphere became increasingly stressful, and it seemed like everyone was on edge all the time. There was a lot of gossiping, backstabbing, and negative interactions between co-workers. The pharmacy was understaffed, and everyone was overworked and underpaid. Despite the work and health challenges, I was happy to serve my patients and ensure that they received the best care possible.

With everything that was going on, I was mad at the world and felt like rebelling. *"How come this is happening to me? How will I be able to help my family if I am not well? How are we going to survive?"*

What I did next was unexpected. I've always been shy, preferring to blend into the background rather than be in the spotlight. But I wanted to do something that for me was insane. In my mind, if I died tomorrow, at least I did something that would make me feel in control of my body again. Amid chaos and frustration, I made a decision that seemed completely out of character. I signed up for a fitness and physique competition (bodybuilding). It was something I had always admired from afar, much like a beauty pageant, but I never thought I could or would participate in it. It was my way of defying the world, of breaking free from the chains that were holding me down.

The fitness competition became my battleground – a place where I could regain a sense of control over my life. It was an act of rebellion against the forces that had sought to break me. I wanted to show the world that I was capable of more and that I would not be confined to the limitations that had been placed upon me.

Little did I know that this decision would change everything. I started to work out and exercise a lot. I changed my eating habits and followed a personalized diet plan. Nutritional supplements were recommended by my trainer to help me with my workouts and to keep my body healthy.

As I trained for the competition, I started to notice changes in my body. My energy levels were higher, and I felt stronger and more empowered. But something else was happening too. The lump in my throat was getting smaller.

At first, I thought it was just my imagination, but when I went back to the doctor for a check-up, they confirmed it. The lump was shrinking. They couldn't believe it. They had never seen anything like it before.

The doctors told me that the combination of diet and exercise had helped my body fight off the lump. They said that I had given my body the tools it needed to heal itself. I did not have to undergo surgery or any other treatment.

I was overjoyed. I had rebelled against my diagnosis, and it had led me to a solution. I went on to compete in the physique competition, and I did well. More importantly, I had taken control of my health, and I had won.

Around this time, I decided to leave the pharmacy and find a new job. It was a difficult decision, but I knew that I needed to prioritize my health and well-being. I found a new job that was a better fit for me, and I noticed a significant improvement in my health and overall happiness.

Now, I continue to follow a healthy lifestyle. I exercise regularly, and I eat a healthy diet. I am grateful for the experience that led me here, and I am thankful for the rebellious spirit that helped me find a solution to my problem.

The Power of Functional Medicine

I discovered the power of Functional Medicine by accident through my health journey and experience of illness. Functional Medicine is a type of holistic healthcare that focuses on treating the root causes of illness, rather than simply masking symptoms with medication. It emphasizes the importance of nutrition, lifestyle, and environmental factors in maintaining health. With my background in pharmacy, I became fascinated with its principles.

As I learned more about "food as medicine," it all started to make sense. I realized that my diet then was filled with processed foods and sugar. I began to experience various health symptoms. My blood pressure was up at a young age, and I developed a lump in my throat. I gained weight, had no energy, and was always tired. I was experiencing the negative health consequences of the Western diet.

The Western diet, also known as the Standard American Diet (SAD), is characterized by high consumption of processed foods, red meat, sugary beverages, refined grains, and unhealthy fats. Unfortunately, this dietary pattern has been linked to numerous negative health effects, contributing to the rise of chronic diseases, obesity rates, and certain types of cancer.

I also believe that part of the health issues I had was due to the constant stress I was experiencing in the workplace. Stress is an intrinsic part of our daily lives, affecting us both physically and mentally. While occasional stress is normal and manageable, chronic stress can have a detrimental impact on our overall health. Particularly concerning is its association with the development and progression of chronic diseases and cancer.

The body's natural stress response, known as the fight-or-flight response, triggers the release of stress hormones like cortisol and adrenaline. When stress becomes chronic, these hormones can disrupt the delicate balance of the body, leading to a variety of health issues.

Functional Medicine was the right choice for me. It gave me the tools I needed to take charge of my health, and I'm grateful for the positive changes it has brought into my life.

The New Mission

As I continued my health transformation, I felt a calling to share my newfound knowledge and experiences with others. My new mission is to contribute to eradicating cancer worldwide through a holistic and Functional Medicine approach, an approach that I wished I knew when I worked as an oncology pharmacist.

I believe that by combining the best of conventional medicine with a natural and holistic approach, we can provide patients with the best possible care and increase their chances of healing.

The integration of conventional medicine with natural and holistic therapies can offer a more comprehensive and personalized approach to patient care. Chemotherapy, radiation, and surgery, while effective, can often cause significant physical and emotional distress. Natural therapies such as herbal remedies, acupuncture, meditation, and nutritional counseling can complement conventional treatments by supporting the immune system, reducing side effects, and promoting overall well-being. This combination can empower patients to take an active role in their healing process. It encourages them to make positive lifestyle changes, such as adopting a healthy diet, engaging in regular exercise, managing stress, and seeking emotional support. These lifestyle modifications can have a profound impact on the outcome of cancer treatment and long-term survivorship.

In 2022, I decided to start my practice, offering holistic cancer care services that complemented traditional treatments. I created my protocols to help clients experience the same holistic healing that I have experienced. Now I can say that my childhood dream came true. I help patients who have cancer find a way to fight and overcome the disease through the power of nutrition and Functional Medicine.

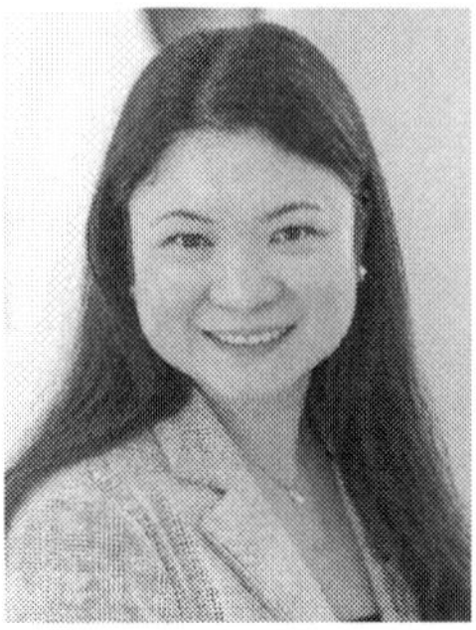

ABOUT JACKIE LYN VELASCO, MS RPH

Jackie Lyn Velasco has been a pharmacist for over 20 years, a Functional Medicine practitioner, and a nutrition and wellness coach. She is the founder and CEO of Purple Nutrition and Wellness™ and Purple Berry Health™, offering nutritional and wellness coaching and functional medicine services to cancer patients or clients at higher risk of developing cancer. She loves to cook, bake and create healthy recipes.

She has served as a faculty member at the College of Pharmacy, University of the Philippines Manila. She trained in clinical oncology pharmacy in Malaysia, Thailand, and Singapore. She helped set up the first Comprehensive Cancer Center Pharmacy at a prestigious tertiary hospital and served hundreds of cancer patients. She was one of the pioneers in the field of Oncology Pharmacy in the Philippines. She has played a significant role in the expansion of oncology pharmacy practice in the country by training other pharmacists in the field of Oncology and has been invited as a guest speaker in various hospitals.

As a pharmacist, she is loved by her patients for her professionalism, compassion, and personalized care.

Jackie believes that her true calling is to use her accumulated knowledge and expertise to help improve and touch as many lives as possible in the holistic healing and prevention of chronic diseases like cancer. Inspired by her health transformation, her mission is to guide, educate and empower many to take control of their health and wellness through the power of nutrition and functional medicine.

"It has never been more relevant to unleash the power within you, take control of your health, and heal the world from diseases like cancer."

– **Jackie Velasco**

www.purpleberryhealth.com | info@purpleberryhealth.com |
www.purplenutritionandwellness.com |
FB/IG/LI: @purplenutritionandwellness
FB/IG/LI: @jackievelascorph

SYNCHING INTO HEALTH: BEGIN TO HEAL THE ENERGY BODY, HEAL THE PHYSICAL BODY

By: Dr. Sadia Yahya,
MD, ABIM, ABIHM, ABFM, CSWWC

"You are not who you think you are."
– Gurudev (Yogi Amrit Desai)

The first step in my healing journey was to reflect on "Who am I?" Once I realized I am not only this physical body or simply a separate entity doomed to watch it fall apart through the natural progression of life and "dis-ease," everything shifted. This all came full circle in February of 2008 when I broke my knee after a bicycle accident. I had already been meditating daily for five years up to that point, and was lucky enough to have met my Guru, my spiritual master, in November of 2007, which brought my practice to a much deeper level. Prior to that, I was very cerebral in my thinking, and had no clue about the healing powers that our own body has waiting for us to tap into.

They say there are no accidents in life, and everything serves as our teacher if we allow it. Around that time, I was interviewing for some temp physician work in an urgent care clinic in Tampa, FL, and the recruiter kept asking if I had been to the local Hindu temple or met a guy named "Gurudev." I was perplexed as to why she kept bringing this up in a medical interview and didn't see the connection. Afterwards, I contemplated the significance of the encounter over my entire drive of one hour. At that point, I decided to listen to the inner guidance that was telling me to go to the weekend seminar she was mentioning, where I would get to meet Gurudev. That weekend seminar blew my rational, scientific, logical "thinking" mind forever. I cannot believe that a broken knee that ensued three months later, after which I had to have major surgery with a cadaver bone graft, two plates, and four screws, would ironically be called a blessing as a teacher and forever change the way that I looked at not only my own body's healing potential but overall healing in general.

This put me on the road to Integrative and Functional Medicine, thereby for once seeing there is something else more out there than what regular allopathic, Western medicine had taught me up until that point in time. We are truly our own healers, with lifestyle factors and choices affecting our very own genes, referred to as "epigenetics." I learned how to tap into the "inner healer" through the deepest meditations that I continued and have continued with daily for over 20 years. I learned how to access that "pranic healing" energy, also known as "chi" or vital life-force energy, to deliver healing and immense pain-relief to my physical body. I began to see the miracles of meditation and the possibilities

of other factors that are there in a holistic sense to aid in our healing journey. At that point forward I was determined to share this empowerment with anyone who came to me.

Also, around that same time, I was struggling with a failing marriage, and I began to develop GI issues with bad acid reflux and stomach pains that were waking me up in the middle of the night. As a doctor, I clearly knew those were "red flag signs." I got in with the GI doctor and my suspicion was correct, that I was developing pre-ulcers known as gastritis. Obviously, I knew that I needed to get out of that toxic relationship, and was of course physically absorbing all the stress, as well. My diet wasn't horrible, but it wasn't optimal either. All the GI doctor offered me were pills to suppress the acid production. When I read about the side effects of the pills, I was in shock: thinning of the bones, decreased magnesium levels, anemia across all the blood lines, and alteration of the gut microbiome, to name a few. I began to think there had to be a better way than simply trying to control the symptoms and actually help to heal the area instead. This also opened a gateway for me to go deeper into Integrative and Functional Medicine to address the root cause of what was going on with me. Through proper diet, nutrition, supplements, and alteration of other factors in my lifestyle, I was able to successfully reverse and cure this issue holistically within the time span of about one year. Of course, it took dedication and persistence, but the results paid off with not having to be on a medication that had a plethora of long-term issues. I was lucky that I did not stay on it, because after my leg had broken, I found out that I had thinning of the bones called osteopenia. The acid-suppressing medicine would have worsened that for sure. Then, my endocrinologist was trying to place me on a medication for osteopenia that I could not tolerate. Luckily, that too I ended up reversing holistically through the proper supplements, exercises, and changes in diet.

We are not meant to watch our bodies turn into a "train wreck" of different ailments. We are not merely the physical body – we are so much vaster than that. Our physical bodies are a gift designed to move toward healing and wholeness if and only if we present them with the optimal circumstances and tools. We are not meant to be victims of "dis-ease." This is when I began to realize the importance of an integrative approach to health, and decided to learn more. In 2016, I became certified in Integrative Holistic Medicine. I went on further in 2021, and became a Diplomat of the American Board of Integrative Medicine after getting grand-fathered into Dr. Andrew Weil's program through all the Integrative Medicine coursework I had been doing through that time.

Through the busy days of working in urgent care for over 10 years, I always found a way to give patients a holistic "pearl" in their treatment. It didn't matter how pressed for time I was, but I always felt I was doing a disservice if I did not offer a holistic or integrative angle in their care. For example, if someone came in with an upper respiratory tract infection, like COVID, I would share a holistic approach to their recovery, including a regimen of supplements, botanicals, and other things for immune support that helped them tremendously. If I saw someone with a pain issue related to an acute injury, I would show them yoga poses to help with their discomfort and advise of dietary changes, supplements, plus other holistic modalities to help decrease their pain.

For the past five years, I have been working at a health and wellness center in a corporate setting. I see people across the gamut with different health issues. I continue to offer holistic pieces of information for their care. I have seen people get off their GI medications or reduce the dosages based on my recommendations for that and other issues. I have helped people with allergies and asthma optimize their care through this functional approach, as well. I have people with anxiety and depression come in with active panic attacks, and I teach them meditation on the spot to clinically reduce their symptoms, with them often leaving like they had a complete makeover, with a smile on their face from cheek to cheek. It is my passion and has been my passion to treat each person by looking at the root cause of their illness and optimizing changes in their life to improve those health issues.

In my childhood, I saw my dad in and out of the hospital for different complications from diabetes. My parents were immigrants who came to the U.S. in the '70s with only $100 in their pockets, and who lived in a cramped room in my aunt's place for a few weeks until they found jobs and could sustain themselves on their own. My dad worked hard, really hard, going to school full-time to pursue his Master's in Business Administration, meanwhile holding three different jobs to support us. I was an observant child, and I decided from a young age that I did not want to end up with the fate of my dad. I was only in middle school or hardly even high school when I became committed to never allowing my genes or family destiny to influence me to develop diabetes. Health class and science were always my favorites. From that age, I began to learn about good nutrition and what we can do to prevent illness. My poor dad developed type 2 diabetes at age 27, which at that time was not common. I remember my mom frequently commented that she would make a whole pot of rice for us for dinner to accompany the curry dish she made, and he would eat almost all of the rice himself. As a child, I had the awareness to realize this couldn't have been good. However, worse than that was the imbalanced life my dad led. I realize now he didn't see any other way, with having limited support in this country and having to make it on his own to support my mom, myself, my brother, and my sister. This observation regarding a balanced life became paramount in my life.

In high school, I realized I wanted to become a doctor and help others to heal. I had little understanding of what allopathic medicine really stood for at that time. Back home, in India and Pakistan, where my family was from, anyone who went to medical school was also trained in

Ayurveda, which is the ancient medical system of the East that our Western medical system is based on, but unfortunately, in modern times it has mutated to a version that is devoid of much of the ancient teachings. This is also why I think I was discouraged with the practice of medicine here in the West. I really wanted to touch back upon the ancient systems. For the first time in our lives, the average life expectancy of Americans has fallen, and we are not leading the world in good-outcome medical statistics for our nation. I think what has been forgotten are the pieces that prevented people from entering into "dis-ease" as we know it today. There is so much more to health and wellness that has been forgotten, and my mission is to reignite that flame to prevent people from developing end-stage issues.

When I went to medical school in the Dominican Republic, my personal scare was having a severe asthma attack that landed me in the ER. Luckily, one of my classmates' moms was there, and she was a registered nurse trained in the U.S. She decided to take me to the ER, which relieved some anxiety about being in an ER in a foreign country. They were about to inject me with something without even telling me what it was. I demanded to know what it was before they administered it, and found out it was theophylline. Right away I thought they must think my asthma is pretty severe if they were going to give me that, because this medicine was a last resort treatment in the U.S., and in fact, it is not on the market anymore due to its severe and even lethal side-effect profile. Later that evening and for the next two days I had trouble walking and was practically paralyzed with severe muscle weakness. I even needed a friend to carry me to the bathroom, which was quite embarrassing. I was about 21 years old at that time and was pretty healthy other than the asthma, which I knew was triggered more due to the heavy pollution there. At that point in time, I also made it part of my mission to find out how to deal with asthma holistically. Later in my journey, I found out about different supplements, environmental factors, specific forms of meditation, and dietary factors that could help diminish outbreaks. They say asthma is increasing in prevalence in the world every year, but they are not sure why. My goal is to help people decrease their outbreaks and be able to breathe better. Our breath is everything and is the beginning of healing. Even in meditation, the focal point of breathing and the pauses between the breath are where we tap into the inner healing potential.

What I have to offer is to help people reach a root cause impact in their lives, as I have done for my own health. The purpose is to help people to reset themselves into their innate state of healing and wholeness before the storm of "dis-ease" has taken them for a long and unnecessary ride. We are the drivers of our own destiny, and once we realize what we can change in our lifestyles, there are many obstacles we can overcome in this healing journey. My goal is to aid people with respiratory and gut issues like asthma or acid reflux to promote their healing on a consulting basis through Functional and Integrative Medicine tools. I will offer HTMA (hair tissue mineral analysis), and help people with pain related to injuries improve their quality of lives through balancing of the mineral ratios in their bodies. Also, I will offer programs that integrate medical meditation into the protocol to help aid in the journey of self-empowerment, as well as, to complement the inner healing work from an energy and mind wellness perspective.

My programs will help people realize they are not on their own in this journey, and also to realize their full potential of wholeness. Remember, we are not the "pain body," and we do not have to accept the pain associated with "dis-ease" as our final destination. We can detour this destination into a place of healing and rebalancing the physical body, so we are no longer victims of ailments. We have been conditioned to feel very fragmented in our own health, but this does not have to be the way anymore. I will help others overcome fear, as I once unknowingly had as an obstacle to healing and feeling better in my own life, and instead embrace a mindset of balance and wholeness.

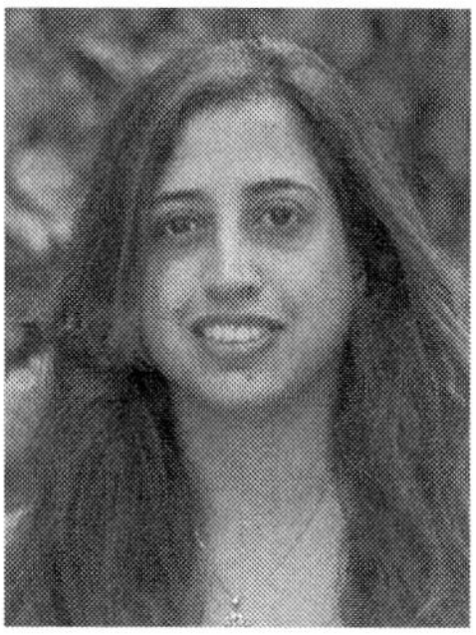

ABOUT DR. SADIA YAHYA,

MD, ABIM, ABIHM, ABFM, CSWWC

Dr. Sadia Yahya is a seasoned medical doctor, turned holistic wellness coach, with over 20 years of experience and a profound commitment to Integrative Medicine and Holistic approaches. Having faced her own health challenges, she understands the limitations of allopathic care and embarked on a journey to explore alternative paths to healing. Her personal experiences with pre-ulcers, life threatening asthma, and reconstructive knee surgery inspired her to pursue certification in Integrative Holistic Medicine. She is a diplomat of the board of Integrative Medicine, Integrative Holistic Medicine, and Family Medicine.

Dr. Yahya firmly believes in the power of proper lifestyle choices, nutrition, and functional medicine tools, combined with mindfulness meditation practices, to foster better breathing, digestion, and overall well-being. She is currently enrolled in STORRIE Institute™ to become a Certified STORRIE Wholistic Wellness Coach™ (CSWWC). Dr. Yahya continues to expand her expertise to offer comprehensive care to her clients.

With over two decades of meditation practice and a yoga teacher certification, she is developing a unique system of medical-based meditation to empower professionals in tuning into their bodies, re-programming breathing and digestion patterns for optimal health. Dr. Yahya's mission is to share her meditation techniques in any program she offers to help others reclaim their health and vitality beginning from the inside-out.

As the owner of "Mindful Holistic Consulting, LLC," Dr. Yahya offers mineral rebalancing for corporate professionals seeking improved breathing, digestion, and faster injury recovery. Her programs include guided Medical Meditation™ sessions, tailored to address individual needs. She will also be offering programs for optimizing gut health.

Passionate about learning, Dr. Yahya regularly attends Holistic Medical Conferences, exploring the potential of supplements and plant medicine. She firmly believes in "food as medicine" and enjoys sharing recipes and herbal teas that promote well-being. Join Dr. Yahya on your path to holistic healing and discover a new state of enhanced well-being.

www.mindfulholisticconsulting.com |
sadiayahya@mindfulholisticconsulting.com |
FB: @mindful solstice consulting

Manufactured by Amazon.ca
Bolton, ON

35919439R00192